D0941541

APPROACH TO ELECTROTHERAPY

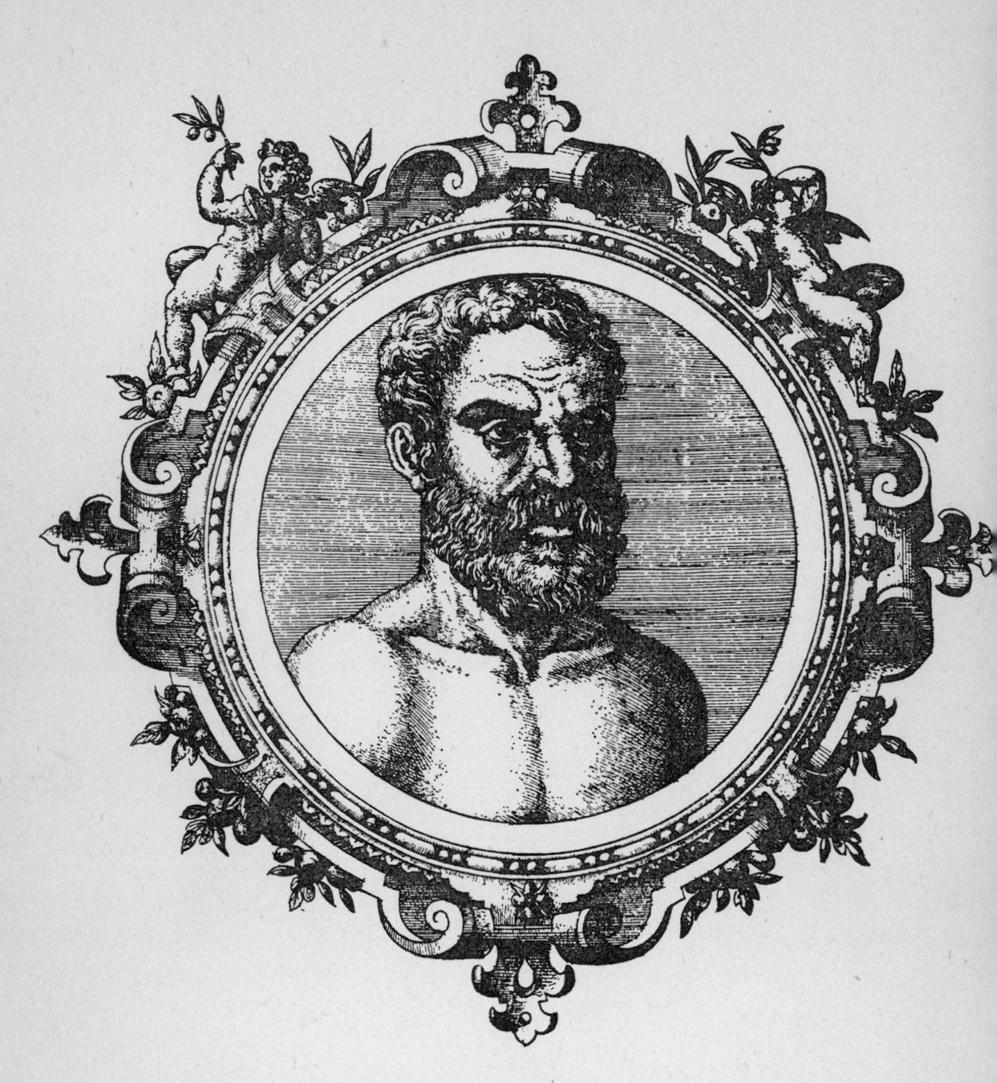

THALES OF MILETUS, 600 B.C.

He discovered that amber, when rubbed, had the property of attracting to itself various light particles. His discovery was the first step in the great science of electricity

Approach to Electrotherapy

BY

R. JEROME LINDQUIST

R. J. Lindquist
2419 WEST NINTH STREET, LOS ANGELES 6, CALIF.
1948

PRINTED BY
ANDERSON & RITCHIE : THE WARD RITCHIE PRESS

CONTENTS

ILLUSTRATIONS

PREFACE

THIS VOLUME is an introduction to the use of modern electrotherapy equipment. In addition to discussing the operation of such equipment, it suggests methods of treatment based on sound and accepted principles of electrophysiology. In other words, it is a statement of the fundamental rules for applying electrical currents to the human body for therapeutic purposes.

An attempt has been made to eliminate as far as possible any suggestion as to how to treat any particular disease or condition. The cases and conditions mentioned are shown as examples only, carefully compiled from the experiences and recommended technics of many specialists. Some general treatment applications are outlined, and from these examples the operator may determine a method of application to fit the case at hand. The prescription of a specific procedure should rest with the specialist in the field of physical medicine.

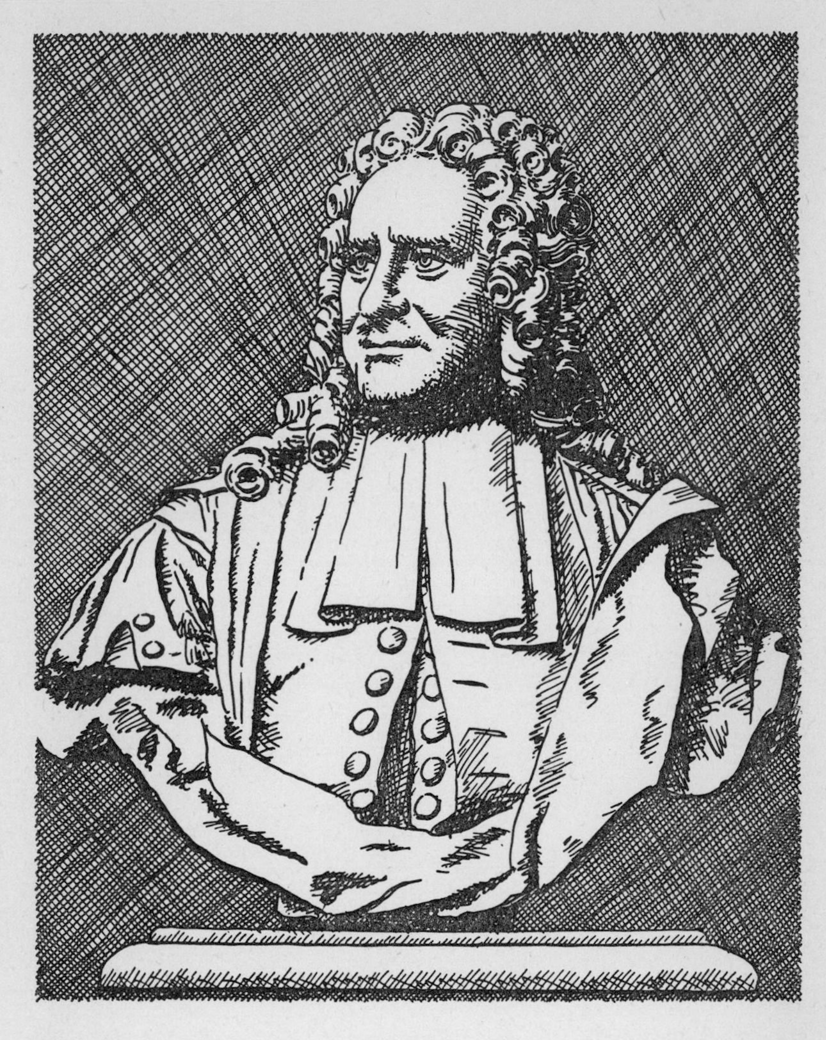

Pieter van Musschenbroek of the University of Leyden (Holland), who about 1745 discovered the Leyden jar, a device for storing charges of static electricity

I
INTRODUCTION TO ELECTROTHERAPY

THE EMPLOYMENT OF ELECTRICITY for therapeutic and diagnostic application to the human body has closely paralleled the development of the use of electricity in many other fields. Early records of experimental electrical devices contain many references to attempts to use electricity in therapy. As early as 1759 a small book entitled "Electricity Made Plain and Useful" appeared in which the author (Wesley) anticipated in theory (and with surprising accuracy) much that has been demonstrated in practice in both electrophysics and electrophysiology.

Most of the early applications were of frictional electricity ("Franklinic" electricity) and made use of the electric bath, electrification by sparks, and shocks from the Leyden jar. The huge static generator with its revolving glass discs, its coated glass jars, and the insulated platform for the patient may still be seen in physics laboratories and in the offices of a few "old timers."

Advances in electrotherapeutics were made possible by three important developments during the nineteenth century. They were (1) the invention of the voltaic pile in 1800, resulting in the introduction of medical and surgical galvanism; (2) Faraday's discovery of the principles of inductive electricity in 1831, and (3) the researches of d'Arsonval toward the end of the century making available the heat-in-tissue-producing properties of high frequency currents.

Present day research in the field of electrotherapy is largely along the lines of identifying the actual physico-chemical processes that activate the body's very complex neuromuscular mechanism, to the end that therapeutic currents of electricity may be better understood in their influence on bodily activity.

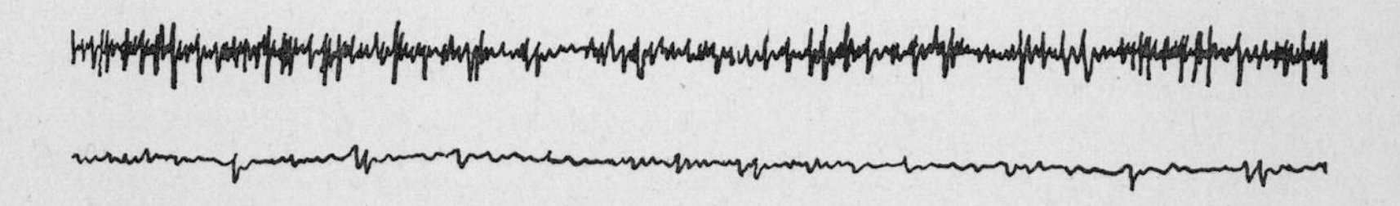

Recordings of electrical potential changes in muscles resulting from muscular activity

DEFINITION. Electrotherapy is a term denoting the use of electricity directly applied to the human body for diagnosis, for alleviation of pain, or for the cure of disease. It includes the use of such remedial measures as short wave diathermy, common ion transfer, galvanism, "sine wave," testing for reaction of degeneration and chronaxy, and various other applications of medical and surgical currents of high and low frequency. The term does not include the use of a great variety of electrically powered apparatus, such as bakers, vibrators, infra-red and ultra-violet lamps, and similar apparatus where electric current is employed as the source of energy without the current's being applied to the body.

VARIETY OF EQUIPMENT. Medical equipment display rooms exhibit for sale a great variety of instruments employing electricity in one form or another. The doctor of today is confronted with a difficult task when he attempts to select, from the diversified equipment offered for sale by therapy manufacturers, instruments best suited to treating his patients. Several questions require consideration:

Is there a physiological response of the patient to the various forms of electrical treatment?

Can pathology or pathological tendencies actually be altered or averted?

Are there specific indications for definite applications?

To be able to answer the above questions intelligently there must first be an elemental basis of understanding that will serve as a common yardstick by which the therapeutic effects of the various devices may be measured. Two methods of analysis may be considered: the electrical and the physiological.

THE ELECTRICAL METHOD. This method requires critical analysis and evaluation on a technical or engineering basis, with detailed study of electrical phenomena, such as direct and alternating currents. Terms such as frequencies, oscillations, harmonics, ergs, ohms, and phases may be confusing to anyone not well grounded in electrical work.

THE PHYSIOLOGICAL METHOD. The physiological approach is the study of the effects of certain commercially available currents and the evaluation of their use solely from responses observed in the living human body. A thorough study of the effects of therapeutic current applications does not require that the technician have a knowledge of electrical engineering. Most technicians prefer to forget the details of the mechanism, leaving that for the engineers;

this enables the technicians to concentrate on the operation of the equipment and the results to be obtained.

In order to simplify and clarify the problems confronting the technician in electrotherapy no attempt will be made to describe in technical detail any of the various types of equipment in use. Observations will be made only about the effects that may be produced, with directions and precautions in their use.

FUNDAMENTAL TYPES OF CURRENTS

There are three fundamental types of electrical current applications, classified according to responses observed when the currents are applied to the body:

1. CHEMICAL EFFECTS. Electrical currents that flow only in one direction produce chemical effects within the tissues immediately adjacent to the areas of application. The ideal form of current producing chemical effects is the galvanic current, which is a constant unidirectional current unwavering in amplitude or intensity. Pulsed or interrupted unidirectional currents also produce chemical effects, but there may be an added contractile effect, depending on the degree to which the flow of current is rippled, or changing rapidly in intensity.

2. CONTRACTILE EFFECTS. Muscular contractions may be produced by short electrical impulses, or currents that are rapidly changing in amplitude. The form of a contractile current may vary within wide limits. It may be sinusoidal, pulsating, interrupted, or oscillatory in type, with a frequency variation anywhere from a few per second to

several thousand per second. It may be nonpolarized or unidirectional. The following are some of the names applied to various types of contractile currents: faradic, sinusoidal, rapid sinusoidal, sine wave, contractive, intermittent, Leduc, static, etc. Since these names often have been applied somewhat loosely, one must remember that all currents with the same name do not necessarily produce identical contractile effects.

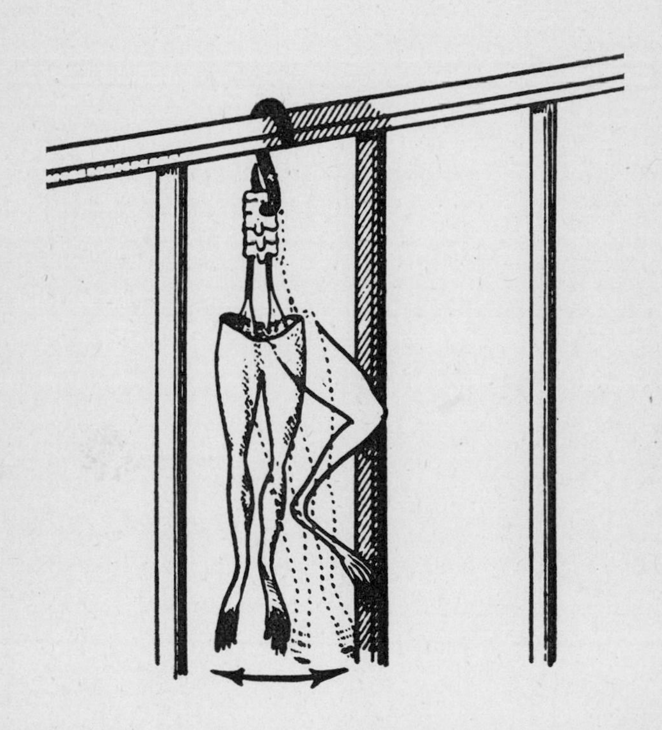

Galvani's "accidental discovery," made when he suspended a frog's legs from an iron balcony in order to dry them. The two dissimilar metals generated an electrical potential, creating a momentary current when wind blew the legs against the metal. Muscular contractions resulted

3. THERMAL EFFECTS. Alternating currents of very high frequency (in excess of 100,000 per second) produce only heating effects. The changes in intensity of each pulsation or alternation take place so rapidly that contractile stimulation of the muscles is not effective. Furthermore, there is no chemical effect because the polarity is completely reversed with each cycle. The entire effect of the passage of high frequency currents through the tissues is the production of heat, which results from the resistance of the tissues to the flow of the electric currents.

In other words, electrical energy transformed from common house-current, when caused to travel in continuous, uninterrupted, unidirectional flow, causes only chemical effects when applied to bodily tissues; the same energy, if rapidly interrupted in flow, or caused to flow in pulses within certain frequency limits, produces only contractile effects; and when caused to flow in extremely high frequency oscillatory current, the effects are entirely thermal. Viewed in this way, it becomes evident that the maximum dosage supplied to the patient by a current of electricity must be gauged by the *effect of the current on the tissue, depending on the type of current employed.* A thorough and complete understanding of this functional control of electrical energy is the key to all successful electrotherapy.

DOSAGE

It is apparent from the foregoing observations that a "therapeutic dose" of electricity differs with the different functions involved. Currents employed for their chemical effects are limited in intensity by the sensation of stinging or mild irritation that is produced in the skin and tissues immediately adjacent to the electrodes, or by the skin reaction immediately following treatment.

If during the application of a galvanic current at somewhere near the maximum intensity that may be comfortably tolerated, the current should suddenly be broken, a single contractile twitch of the muscles involved in the treatment area would result. A similar stronger twitch would result from the sudden restoration of the current flow. If the current were to be broken and restored at a rapid rate (many times per second) a cumulative contractile effect would result from the rapid sequence of make-and-break impulses, with intense tetanic contraction of the muscles, and the current would appear to be too strong to be comfortably tolerated by the patient. The intensity would have to be reduced. The most satisfactory guide to the intensity of contractile currents is the degree of contraction produced in the muscles being stimulated.

In the application of currents employed for their thermal effects no chemical or contractile effects are encountered, and comparatively much greater intensities of electrical energy can be comfortably tolerated by the patient. Why is there such a difference in physiological tolerance? A few milliamperes of contractile current may be all that the patient can tolerate. With the same electrode application, the patient may be able to tolerate 30 or 40 milliamperes of chemical energy. The limit of endurance of thermal energy may be several thousand milliamperes of current. Obviously electrical units do not necessarily coincide with physiological units. A study of the effects of the different forms of electrical currents used in therapy should be based on physiological considerations rather than electrical units. The different effects produced all originate from the same source of energy, generally the 60-cycle alternating lighting supply current, but by means of various appliances the nature of the current is transformed in order to accentuate one or more of the inherent properties of the current.

Graph of a galvanic current

GALVANISM. The galvanic current is an unidirectional current from which all ripples or irregularities have been removed, therefore it is not referred to as having frequency. It varies in amplitude only when turned off or on, or when it is supplied in slowly changing rhythmic surges by the generating mechanism. Such rhythmic changes in intensity are too slow to cause contractile effects, except when used on denervated muscles.

The term "direct current" is not always synonymous with galvanism, because commercial direct current may be composed of a rapid sequence of unidirectional pulses, or ripples. Full-wave rectified house current of 60 cycles produces direct current with a frequency of 120 impulses per second, and is strong in contractile power unless it is filtered. The galvanic current is a direct current that has been well filtered.

CONTRACTILE CURRENTS. A necessary characteristic of a contractile current is that it must be rapidly changing in amplitude, with the change from zero to maximum intensity of each individual pulse of the current taking place within a time of not more than a few hundredths of a second. It is not necessary that the individual impulses of the current be sinusoidal in form. They may be instantaneous

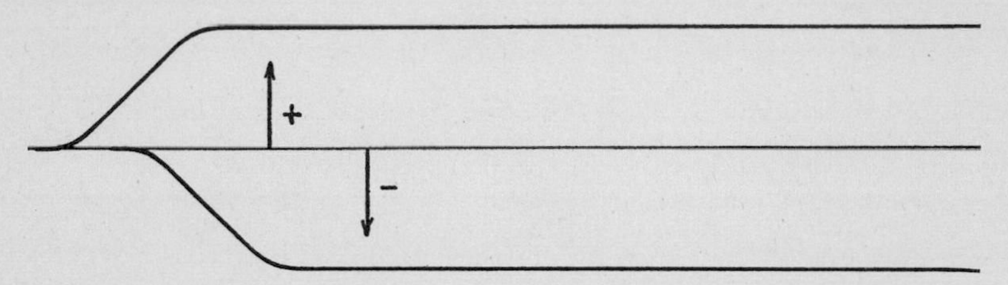

A galvanic current may have positive or negative polarity, depending on direction of flow

makes and breaks of a direct current, or they may be very short "spike" impulses, a rapid sequence of which makes up the familiar faradic current. A wide range of frequencies, and types of "action units" are capable of producing muscular contractions, but all the factors of frequency, intensity, duration, and rate of change in amplitude of the individual impulses making up a current have an important influence on the type of muscular contraction elicited.

POLARITY. The therapeutic effect of an electric current is controlled by the *rate of change* in amplitude of the current. When the rate of change is too slow to elicit a muscular contractile response, the current predominates in electrolytic or chemical effects. The current is then said to have negative or positive polarity, depending on the direction of flow, with different effects at each pole. If the current is slowly reversed, the observed effects will change position at the electrodes, and the polarity is said to be reversed. If the reversal takes place before sufficient time has elapsed to produce much chemical change, the polarity effects will be largely nullified. As the rapidity with which the polarity is reversed is gradually increased, muscular contractions begin to take effect.

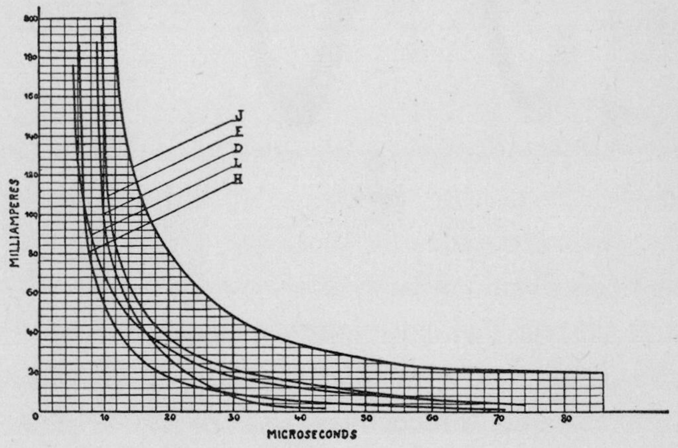

Characteristic frequency-intensity curves obtained from variable frequency stimulation of normal muscles

The contractile effect begins to become effective as the frequency of the polarity change approaches 10 per second for the complete cycle (if the current is sinusoidal in form), and the contractile power continues to increase with the rising frequency until the maximum effect is reached somewhere above 100 cycles per second. As the frequency approaches 3,000 cycles per second the contractile power of the current decreases, and by the time a frequency of approximately 30,000 to 75,000 cycles per second is reached no further contractile effect remains.

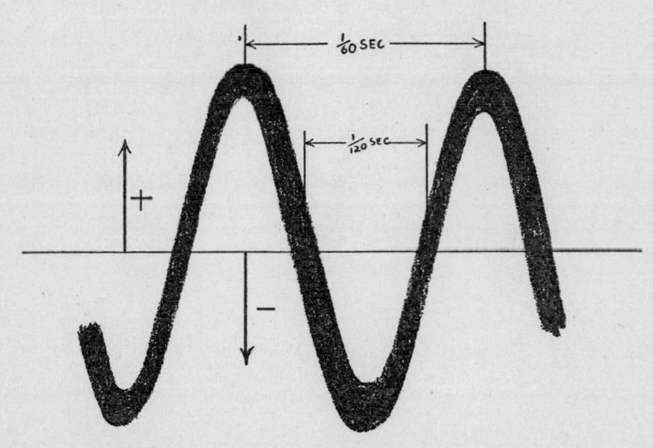

Oscillogram of 60-cycle house current

That the contractile effects are due to the *rate of change* and not to galvanic polarity is shown by the fact that if a galvanic current (which is entirely chemical in its effects) is suddenly rippled, with a frequency of 60 cycles per second, for example, the chemical current instantly takes on the added power of causing muscular contraction. This results in a *combination current*, with the contractile effect added to the chemical effect. Such a current is variously called direct, rippled galvanic, pulsating galvanic, or superimposed.

THERMAL CURRENTS. Diathermy currents, as currents producing thermal effects are called, are of extremely high frequency, 100,000 cycles per second and higher, with alternating polarity every half-cycle. Neither chemical nor contractile effects are produced by diathermy currents.

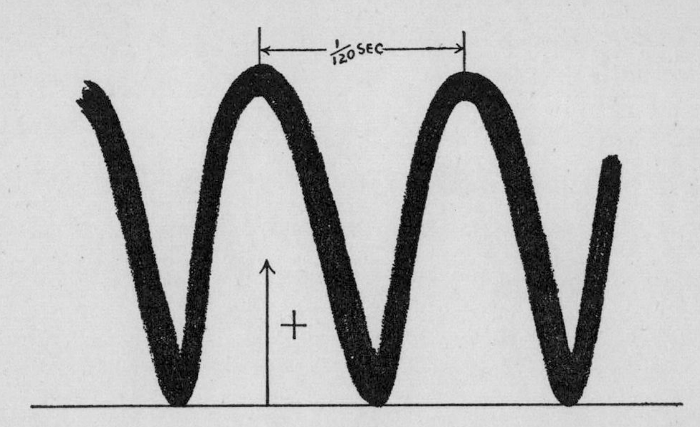

Oscillogram of rectified current, unfiltered, 120 pulsations per second

Each cycle is completed so quickly that no contractile stimulation is possible, and the only effect of the passage of the current through the tissues is the heating effect. The maximum dosage is determined by the maximum heating of the tissues that can be tolerated.

A patient can comfortably tolerate thermal (high frequency) energy in amounts which supplied as chemical energy (galvanism) would cause severe electrolytic destruction or chemical burn over the same area. Likewise, the maximum amount of chemical energy that might comfortably be tolerated, if supplied as efficient contractile energy, would produce intolerable tetanizing or shocking effect. It is possible for a patient to tolerate perhaps 100 times more thermal energy than chemical energy, and in turn he may be able to tolerate only 1/100th as much of certain types of contractile energy as he could comfortably take of galvanism.

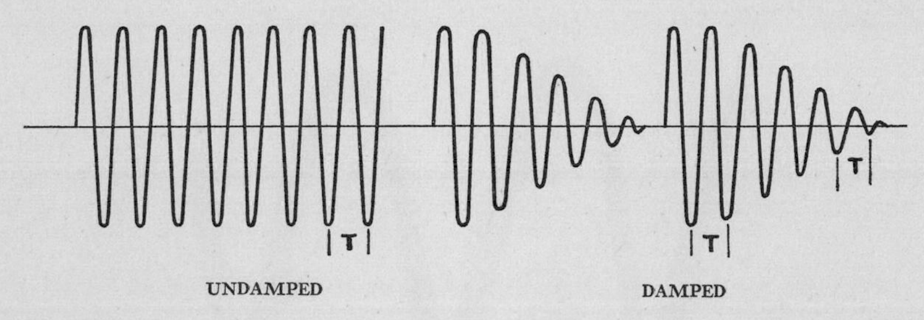

Diagram of high frequency currents. T=1/1,000,000th second or less

Maximum dosages of electrical current that can be tolerated by a patient:

Contractile currents: 1 ma. to 25 ma., depending on frequency, type of "action unit," size of electrode, and sensitivity of part being stimulated.

Chemical currents: 10 ma. to 100 ma., dosage being limited by skin burn sensation and electrolytic action.

Thermal currents: 5,000 to 10,000 ma., the amount being limited only by the rise in temperature of the parts of the body receiving treatment.

The above illustrates the difficulty encountered in measuring intensity of electrical treatments by meter only, without regard to the physiological action of the current.

EXPERIMENTS

AND

OBSERVATIONS

ON

ELECTRICITY,

MADE AT

PHILADELPHIA IN AMERICA,

BY

BENJAMIN FRANKLIN, L.L.D. and F.R.S.

Member of the Royal Academy of Sciences at Paris, of the Royal Society at Gottingen, and of the Batavian Society in Holland, and President of the Philosophical Society at Philadelphia.

To which are added,

LETTERS AND PAPERS

ON

PHILOSOPHICAL SUBJECTS

The Whole corrected, methodized, improved, and now collected into one Volume, and illustrated with COPPER PLATES.

THE FIFTH EDITION

LONDON:

Printed for F. NEWBERY, at the Corner of St. Paul's Church-Yard.

M.DCC.LXXIV.

The name of greatest interest to Americans in connection with early electrical experiments is that of Benjamin Franklin (1706-1790). He attempted to treat patients with shocks from the Leyden jar

II
CHEMICAL EFFECTS

IT HAS BEEN SHOWN that when an electric current flowing preponderantly in one direction is applied to the body the effect of the passage of that current through the tissues is largely chemical in nature. The ideal current to produce such effects is one which in addition to flowing in one direction only is constant and unwavering in intensity, and can be turned slowly on or off as needed. Such a current is generally known as a galvanic current, and its application to the body is known as galvanism.

Indications for the use of galvanism in therapy are many, but before an attempt is made to show some of the more popular uses for the galvanic current a few general observations about the production and control of the chemical effects of electric currents are offered.

THERAPEUTIC ACTION. The chief therapeutic action of the galvanic current is due to the reflex action resulting from the electrolytic stimulation of the cutaneous and subcutaneous nerves immediately beneath the areas over which the current is applied. By this reflex stimulation the valuable sequence of effects of an increased blood supply is obtained.

This stimulation is very similar in nature to what has been termed "counter-irritation," with the great advantage that the amount of stimulation is capable of exact regulation, and that it takes place largely within the epidermis, thus acting directly on the nerve endings. It can be con-

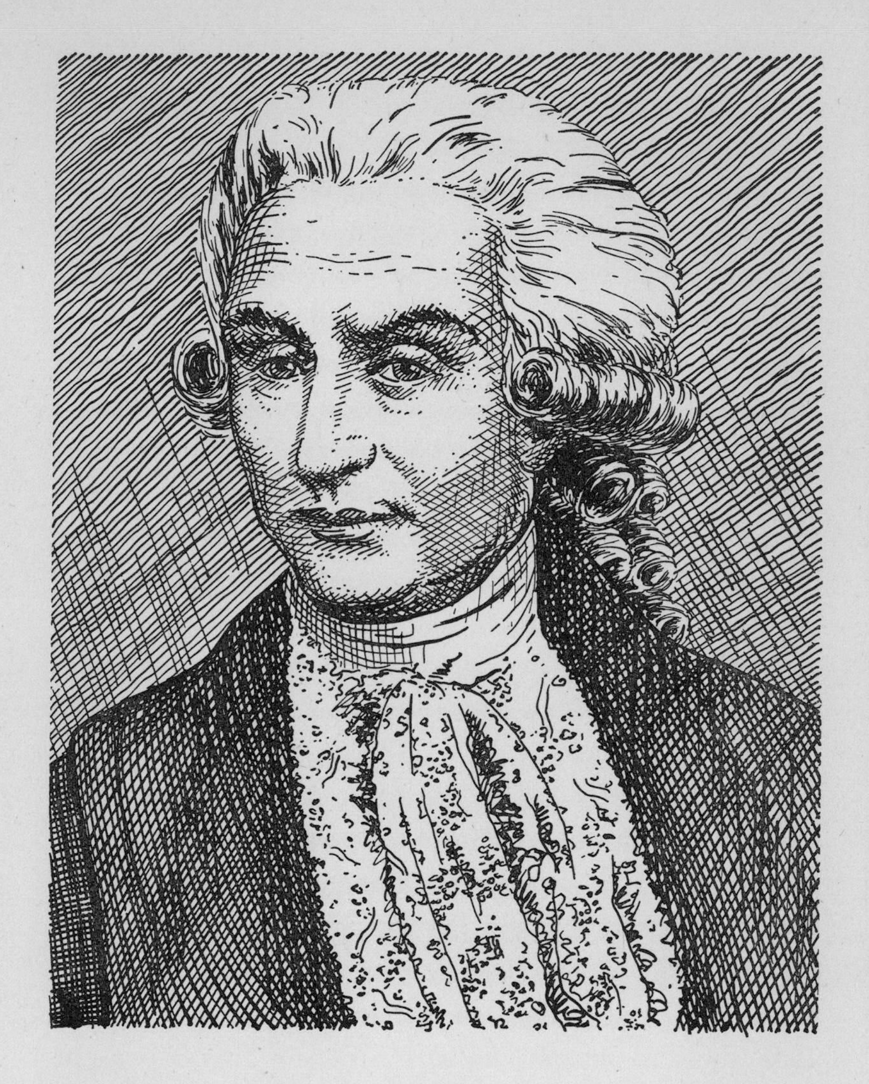

Luigi Galvani (1737-1798), an Italian physician who thought he discovered electricity in animal matter, and from whose name the word galvanism is derived

tinued for as long as several weeks with repeated applications, improving the condition of the skin rather than destroying it, as the constant painting on of an irritant might do. The extent of this stimulation is dependent on the strength and duration of the current employed, the nature of the solutions with which the conducting pads are moistened, and the polarity at which the solution is applied.

When the positive electrode consists of zinc or copper (or salts of these metals in solutions), a caustic and destructive compound such as the chlorides or oxychlorides of the metals is formed in the submucous or subcutaneous area by the combination of zinc or copper ions proceeding from the positive pole to the tissues, and chlorine ions proceeding from the tissues to the positive pole. This method may be valuable for the safe destruction of diseased membranes of cavities, such as the uterus, or the lining of septic cavities.

Similarly, by reducing dosages, or employing milder solutions, a reflex stimulation to the tissues can be accomplished. The amount of stimulation depends on (a) the nature of the solution, and (b) the strength and duration of the current. In general the best results are obtained from the solutions that have the least irritating properties, and the application of current in such strength that it can be tolerated as long as 40 minutes by the patient.

All the tissues of the body conduct electrical energy to a varying degree, the medium of conduction being the fluid of the body. This fluid may be regarded as a combination of several salt solutions (electrolytes). Current is transmitted in the fluid through the migration of ions. When current is applied to the body through an electrolytic conductor, the body and both electrodes should be regarded as three rows of electrical conductors between which ions are exchanged.

GALVANIC TERMS. Many terms have been devised to denote some phase of the electrolytic process involved in the applications of the galvanic current: ionization, electrophoresis, cataphoresis, medical galvanism, and common ion transfer. Ion transfer seems to be gaining in favor as the word best suited to describe many galvanic technics. Surgical galvanism is a term applied to any process where the galvanic current is of such intensity that actual destruction of the tissues adjacent to the electrodes is accomplished.

DEPTH OF IONIC PENETRATION. The question of just how deep ion penetration may go into the tissues is important, because there must be no possibility of producing deep-seated destruction within the tissues. In spite of many claims that have been made for deep penetration of electrically induced ions, it is doubtful that very many ions are introduced deeper than the outer strata of the body. Ion transfer is essentially an intradermal form of treatment, and systemic effects are rare except with the use of certain drugs of high potency, effective when absorbed in very small dosages. Galvanic ionization effects may last for hours, for the skin acts as a reservoir of the drug, which is absorbed later. Some ions (iodine, for example) undoubtedly have greater penetration than others. A few substances, such as histamine, may produce a very strong skin reaction.

PHYSIOLOGICAL CONSIDERATIONS. The galvanic current has two important physiological effects, according to which pole is applied. If two small electrodes are attached to a portion of the body, connected to the positive and negative poles respectively, and a galvanic current is turned on, certain chemical effects occur adjacent to each electrode. First of all, at the negative electrode there would be a liberation of hydrogen, and the litmus reaction would be alkaline. At the positive electrode oxygen would be liberated, but probably this active element would not be noticed since it would unite with the metal of the electrode, or oxidize some of the tissue at the site. Some of the observations may be summarized as follows:

POLARITY EFFECTS OF THE GALVANIC CURRENT

Negative pole	*Positive pole*
Vasodilation	Vaso-constriction
Liberates hydrogen	Liberates oxygen
Liquefies, softens tissue	Dries, hardens tissue
Soft scar	Hard, unyielding scar
More painful (irritant)	Less painful (sedative)
Attracts alkalies	Attracts acids
Promotes hemorrhage	Stops hemorrhage
Relaxes tissue	Contracts tissue
Relieves pain in chronic conditions by increasing circulation	Relieves pain in acute conditions by reducing congestion
Deposits electro-negative ions	Deposits electro-positive ions
More powerful contractions on "make"	Less powerful contractions on "make"

ION TRANSFER. Ions of medical substances can be introduced into the body through the skin and mucous surfaces by taking advantage of the distinctive properties of each pole. Ions with a positive charge are introduced into the tissues from the positive pole (examples: metals, alkaloids). Negatively charged ions (such as iodine, chlorine, and acid radicals) are introduced by the negative pole.

If doubt exists as to the correct pole at which to apply a certain electrolyte, reference should be made to its chemical formula, for the electropositive atoms are always listed first. For example, from the formula for potassium iodide KI we see that potassium ions are applied at the positive pole, iodine ions at the negative pole.

COMMONLY USED SUBSTANCES, WITH POLAR APPLICATIONS

Ion	*Solution*	*Pole*
Zinc	Zinc sulphate	Positive
Copper	Copper sulphate	Positive
Histamine	Histamine chloride	Positive
Choline	Mecholyl	Positive
Iodine	Potassium iodide	Negative
Chlorine	Sodium chloride	Negative
Salicylate	Sodium salicylate	Negative

MOIST ELECTRODES NECESSARY. The dry skin is a poor conductor of electricity and therefore all applications of galvanic currents should be made with the skin well moistened. Electrodes should be well moistened throughout the treatment and should make especially good and uniform contact with the skin. They may be moistened with water or a solution of the drug or chemical to be used. If distilled water is used a small amount of salt should be added to improve conductivity.

IONS IN THE BODY. The galvanic current may also influence the dispersal and concentration of ions already in the body. It is possible, because of this fact, that the simple passage of the unidirectional current through the body may have its greatest therapeutic effect.

IMMEDIATE EFFECTS. The immediate effect produced on the skin next to the electrodes is mainly an increased sensitivity, and a prickling, possibly a mild burning sensation, occurs. This reaction may last for quite some time after the treatment is terminated, and the degree of irritation is in proportion to the intensity and duration of current flow.

INTRADERMIC TREATMENT. Since ions can not be made to migrate very far below the surface of the skin or mucous membranes in any large number, ion transfer is essentially an intradermic form of treatment. For best results the following facts should be noted: (1) inorganic ions from the contact electrodes will travel better than organic ones; (2) weak solutions are better than concentrated solutions; and (3) there must be sufficient time and strength of the galvanic current. For the introduction of drugs it is often advisable to make special applicators for each treatment, to eliminate the possibility of contaminating the standard electrode pads. Blotting paper may be moistened with the solutions to be used and applied directly to the skin, with flexible metal backing, such as tinfoil, making the contact with the current source.

MUCOUS SURFACES. For treatment of mucous surfaces such as cervix, nasal cavity, etc., special metallic electrodes of proper size and shape, or a packing containing the solution with the desired ions, are placed in direct contact with the walls of the cavity, and serve as the active electrode.

VASODILATING DRUGS. Interest in histamine and other vasodilating drugs for improving peripheral circulation in rheumatism, arthritis, and other conditions led to the discovery that when administered by ionization these drugs are readily absorbed, with well-controlled local and systemic effects following the treatment.

APPARATUS. The simplest galvanic apparatus consists of an electric battery, made up of a number of individual cells in series, with a variable resistance to control the intensity of the current from zero to maximum. A meter, calibrated in milliamperes, is almost a necessity, for the reaction of the patient is not a dependable guide to the current intensity. Motor generator sets, too, are in general use, and they are equipped with filter arrangements to smooth out the current flow and to eliminate the contraction-producing pulsations that would otherwise be present. More recently house-current rectifying devices similar to the power packs of radio receivers have been very popular.

SURGING GALVANISM. Some instruments provide a means of surging the galvanic current, in several instances with a complete reversal of polarity with each surge. In every type of instrument it is necessary to employ a rheostat or current control device of sufficient capacity so that the current may be increased or decreased in easy stages without jumps or irregularities, which might cause muscular contractions or shocks to the patient.

METHODS OF APPLICATION

There are three generally used methods of making contact with the body and thus completing the circuit so that galvanic energy may be applied:

1. MOIST PAD ELECTRODES. These consist of flexible metal dispersal plates, covered with absorbent material, such as linen, felt, cotton, or asbestos, and sufficiently thick to distribute the current uniformly to the surface of the skin. Electrodes should be available in a variety of sizes so that all necessary applications can be made. The solution held in suspension by the absorbent material conducts the current from the metal plate of the electrode to the skin.

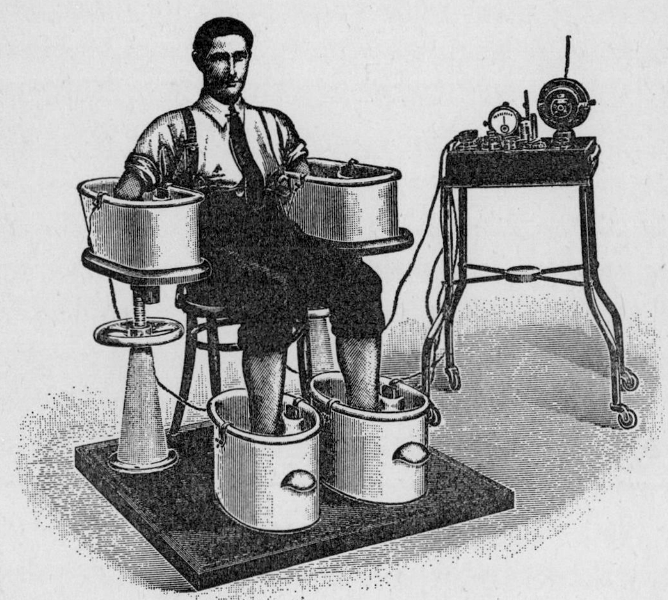

Multiple cell bath (galvanic)

2. CELL BATHS. By this method the limbs or parts of the body to be treated are immersed directly in the electro-

lyte, in tanks, trays, or basins filled with the solution, and the current is passed from the solution to the body.

3. BARE METAL ELECTRODES. These are employed chiefly upon mucous surfaces within the natural cavities, or inserted into tissue by needle puncture. The positive pole attacks and decomposes most metals, except platinum and gold. Carbon may also be used for some types of orificial electrodes.

CARE OF ELECTRODES. Most applications of galvanism are made with moist pad electrodes. The pads should be examined carefully from time to time and should be replaced when decomposition due to electrolytic action is in evidence. The pads should be thoroughly and uniformly moistened with mild saline solution, and they should be sterilized regularly. For sanitary reasons an extra layer of moist cloth or paper should be placed between the moist pad electrode and the skin.

RULES. The following points should be observed in making surface electrode applications

1. The size and shape of the active electrode should be determined according to the area to be treated.

2. The indifferent (dispersive) electrode should be at least equal to and preferably greater in size than the active electrode.

3. Do not treat with greater current intensity than one milliampere per square inch of active electrode area. A safe treatment rule is to keep the current intensity at not more than one half this amount.

INTRODUCTORY TREATMENT. When a patient is being

treated for the first time it might be well to explain briefly the nature of the treatment and the sensations to be experienced. It is not uncommon for patients to be fearful of "electric shock," and they are unable to relax unless mentally prepared. The part to be treated should be well supported, to avoid fatigue, and the patient should be made comfortable. Blankets, bath towels, and rubber sheeting should be provided if necessary to keep the patient's clothing dry. The skin of the areas to be in contact with both the active and the inactive electrodes should be examined carefully. All traces of oils, ointments, liniments, or other applications, when found, should be carefully removed with alcohol, or with soap and water. Foreign substances may increase the possibility of skin burns. If abrasions are found they should be covered with dry gauze and adhesive tape.

Electrodes of the proper size and shape should be applied only after being thoroughly soaked in weak saline solution. They should be bound firmly in place, or supported snugly with pressure in such a way as to make firm and uniform contact. A perfect contact is necessary to prevent spotted current concentration.

PREPARING THE INSTRUMENT. Make sure that all switches of the apparatus are turned off before the patient's lead cords are connected to the electrodes. Examine all wires and connections to see that contacts are secure. Check the polarity-changing switch to see that the polarity of the active electrode is correct for the solution to be ionized. The power control should be set at zero before the instrument is turned on, or before the polarity switch is changed.

STARTING TREATMENT. To start the treatment the current should be turned on by *slowly* advancing the power control knob (rheostat). If a stinging sensation is felt by the patient it might be well to wait a few minutes before advancing the power to the predetermined intensity, as shown by the milliammeter. In any case of excessive burning or painful sensation, the current should be turned off slowly, and the patient's skin re-examined for possible abrasions, or the electrodes checked for insufficiently moistened pads, or faulty contact.

When the current is to be applied for a period longer than 20 minutes it is sometimes necessary to moisten the electrodes again to prevent excessive skin irritation.

At the end of the time prescribed the current should be turned gradually and completely off. The electrodes may now be removed, the patient's skin dried and examined, and possibly dusted with talcum powder. There should be no more than a slight redness of the skin under the electrodes, and a slight feeling of warmth in the areas treated, except when histamine and similar drugs have been used (from which a more intense reaction is anticipated). If burns should be produced they are the result of metal touching the skin during treatment. They will never occur if careful technic is employed.

TESTS FOR POLARITY. If there is any doubt about the polarity of the galvanic current, a quick test may be made in either of the following ways:

1. Immerse the two cord tips in a tumbler of water, with the terminals about 1 inch apart. Turn on about 20 ma. of

current. The tip that shows the formation of the greatest number of bubbles is the *negative* pole.

2. Grasp a treatment electrode in each hand. Turn on about 5 to 8 ma. of current or more if necessary, and then change the position of the polarity switch. The hand that receives the sharpest contractile impulse is connected to the *negative* pole.

SUMMARY OF TREATMENT PRECAUTIONS IN GALVANIC APPLICATIONS

1. Patients should experience little, if any, sensation during treatment. A slight tingling is all that is permissible.

2. Watch carefully for abrasions, and cover them.

3. Check all contacts carefully *before* starting treatment.

4. The current must be turned on *slowly*, the patient being watched for possible distress. Turn current off with equal care.

5. Anesthetic and scar areas must be treated with extreme care.

6. If adjustment of electrodes is necessary, the current should first be turned off slowly and completely.

7. Any erythema or slight reddening or increased sensitivity of the skin should be allowed to subside before further treatment. To produce the best results the galvanic current must be administered with carefully selected and individualized technic.

SOLUTIONS FOR IONIC MEDICATION. The solutions for ionizations may be prepared in advance and kept in stock solutions to be diluted at the time of use. A dilution of two per cent may be used in most instances, except substances which are painful of introduction, such as zinc chloride, when 1% is of sufficient strength. Histamine may be used in solutions weaker than 1/10th of 1%.

Zinc solution: zinc sulphate, 75 grains; glycerine, 2 ounces; water, 35 ounces. Dilute one half when using.

Zinc gelatin: zinc sulphate, 8.75 grains; gelatin, 65 grains; water, 1 ounce.

Sodium salicylate solution: sodium salicylate, 175 grains; water, 1 pint. Dilute one half when using.

Iodine: potassium iodide, 2%.

THE ANTISEPTIC IONS. The following ions may be employed for their antiseptic properties: zinc, copper, mercury, silver, and chlorine. The metals are applied at the positive pole, chlorine at the negative.

A few of the other ions that have been used are quinine, calcium, magnesium, cocaine, adrenalin, aconite, and thiosinamin, applied at the positive pole; and sulphur, chromium, fluorine, oxygen, and phosphorus, applied at the negative pole.

REPRESENTATIVE GALVANIC TECHNICS

MEDICAL GALVANISM. Moist pad electrodes are placed adjacent to the areas to be treated, and current strength is kept well below the patient's tolerance. Treatments may be from 10 to 40 minutes in duration, with intensities as high as 20 to 30 ma. The pads are moistened with water (slightly saline), and no attempt is made to introduce additional ions into the body through the skin.

Medical galvanization may be employed in (1) rheumatism and chronic arthritis, (2) inflammation resulting from traumatism, contusions, and myositis, (3) neuritis and neuralgia, and (4) chronic circulatory disturbances, such as neurasthenia.

The treatment is based on the theory that galvanic current applied to a part of the body surface causes vasomotor stimulation of the skin and increased circulation and nutrition of the parts in the path of the current. This speeds up the resolution of the inflammatory products, and the resultant relief of pressure relieves pain. This treatment may be applied by means of the galvanic cell baths.

ION TRANSFER. The same general technic is followed in ionization as that used in medical galvanism, except that strict attention is paid to the polarity of the active electrode. Special solutions are employed for specific effects, and it is important that the correct pole be employed. Blotting paper may be moistened with the drug solution and applied directly to the skin, with moist gauze or asbestos pad over the paper. The dispersive electrode is soaked only in saline solution.

HISTAMINE IONIZATION. Due to the intensely irritating quality of histamine, treatment intensities and duration are less than with most ionizing solutions. Use 1/1000 solution, ½ ma. per square inch, 3 to 5 minutes, positive pole.

The resulting skin reaction often results in an itching sensation and the formation of definite wheals on the skin. Sometimes the reddening extends beyond the area of the electrodes. There is a rise in temperature of the treated area. The reddening disappears within a few hours.

MECHOLYL. Mecholyl ionization is used in arthritis and circulatory disturbances. This compound is described as the antagonist of adrenalin. It is applied at the positive pole, 1% solution, 15 to 30 ma., 10 to 20 minutes. It is contraindicated where there is fever, or for patients who have bronchial or other types of asthma. It must be used with caution in cases of heart involvement. Its use includes peripheral vascular pathologies, including Raynaud's disease.

EAR INFECTIONS. Zinc ionization has been used in uncomplicated middle-ear suppuration, especially with large drum perforation. The canal and middle ear are carefully cleansed with cotton applicators wet with 1% zinc sulphate solution. Then with the patient lying on the opposite side, the ear and canal are filled with the same solution. The positive pole of the galvanic current is connected by means of a zinc wire electrode to the solution-saturated cotton in the ear, protected by means of a glass or rubber speculum. Current strength is 2 to 3 ma., 10 to 15 minutes. Two treatments per week may be given safely. If auditory nerve disturbance follows the treatment, it is sometimes relieved by the application of faradic current at tolerance, for 5 minutes.

ZINC IONIZATION FOR RHINITIS AND HAY FEVER. After anesthetization, the nasal cavity is filled by packing with slender pledgets of cotton wet with 1% zinc sulphate solution, or with zinc jell. The olfactory area of the upper nose must not be so packed, or anosmia may result. A slender zinc wire is wrapped lightly in cotton and is introduced between the inferior turbinate and the septum. The wire must penetrate the pack almost its entire length, but the bare wire must not touch the tissues. Apply the positive pole, to a tolerance not exceeding 10 ma., for 10 to 15 minutes. Pain, similar to neuralgia, may follow for a period of eight to twelve hours.

COPPER IONIZATION OF CERVIX. A set of Tovey electrodes is recommended, with tips of various sizes. A series of negative galvanic applications, with slightly larger dilating electrodes each succeeding treatment, will soften the tissue and dilate the canal preceding copper ionization. The largest copper electrode that can be passed should be used for the final treatment, 15 to 30 ma., for 20 to 30 minutes, causing a chemical coagulation of the membranes lining the canal. Reduce current to zero, reverse polarity, and apply negative current for an additional three to five minutes in order to insure against membranes' adhering to electrode.

SCARS. Use 1% solution of sodium chloride, or potassium iodide, on a thick pad making good contact with the scarred area. Use current intensity of 5 to 30 ma., depending on the size of the area treated, for 30 minutes. Daily treatments may be given. Satisfactory results have been reported where treatment has been continued over a period of several weeks.

ENDOMETRITIS. Copper or zinc metallic electrodes are used, with a dosage ranging from 10 to 25 ma., for 15 to 30 minutes. After the positive treatment the polarity must be reversed in order to withdraw the electrode.

HEMORRHOIDS, RECTAL PROLAPSUS. A copper electrode is used, positive pole, 10 to 15 ma., 10 to 15 minutes. Best results are obtained with the electrode covered with gauze or chamois and saturated with 2% copper sulphate.

REMOVAL OF SUPERFLUOUS HAIR (EPILATION). A sufficient strength of current (.5 to 2 ma.) is applied by means of thin needles inserted into the hair follicle to destroy the follicular lining, the papilla, and the hair root. If properly carried out, this treatment is followed by a smooth and almost invisible scar and the total disappearance of the unwanted hair. The negative pole is employed.

REMOVAL OF MOLES AND WARTS. Because of the safety of the method and excellent cosmetic results, many men prefer the galvanic method, although the high frequency method is now largely used for the destruction of superficial growths. Skin conditions that may be successfully treated with electrolysis are moles with hair, rosacea, spider nevus, angioma of small size, filiform and flat warts, and adenoma sebaceum.

HEMORRHOIDS—KEESEY METHOD. A specially constructed steel needle with an insulated shaft is used as the active electrode from the negative pole. The needle is inserted in the longitudinal axis of the lumen of the hemorrhoidal vein, care being taken not to transfix it. Needles with different-length tips are available, so the correct size can be selected. Each has a finely tapered edge of the insulating shaft, so that the hydrogen gas generated at the tip of the needle will not be permitted to escape.

A current of 10 to 15 ma. is applied for 5 to 10 minutes until the entire tumor turns dark red or black in color. Following the treatment, the thrombosed mass is absorbed with very little pain. Large hemorrhoids should be treated about every third day, separate parts of the tumor being treated with a current flow of not more than five minutes after the first application. Keesey estimates about six treatments are required for the average large mass, and it is claimed that recovery is smooth, hemorrhage never occurs, and recurrence is rare. This method is for internal hemorrhoids only.

ULCERS. Zinc sulphate with the positive pole, or potassium iodide with the negative pole, is used, with a strength of 1 to 3 ma. per square inch, 10 to 20 minutes duration.

COPPER IONIZATION FOR FUNGUS. Treatment is made by placing the extremity in a cell bath, in which it is immersed in 1% copper sulphate. The positive pole is used, 15 to 25 ma., 15 to 30 minutes. To insure uniform distribution of the current, the skin should not come in direct contact with the copper electrode used to distribute the current through the solution. The negative electrode is placed on the upper part of the leg.

PARALYSIS. The galvanic current in therapeutic dosages seldom produces contractions. In some cases this fact has led to the erroneous belief that galvanism is of no value in the treatment of paretic muscles. Although actual contractions of the muscles may not be produced, the excitability of the muscles is increased, and local increase in temperature follows the treatment. This hyperemia may be very pronounced, and involves not only the skin, but also the subjacent layers.

The treatment examples given here are indicative of the wide range of therapeutic applications that may be made, using the galvanic current for its chemical effects on the tissues of the body. Additional uses of the galvanic current are suggested in the treatment chart for low voltage currents.

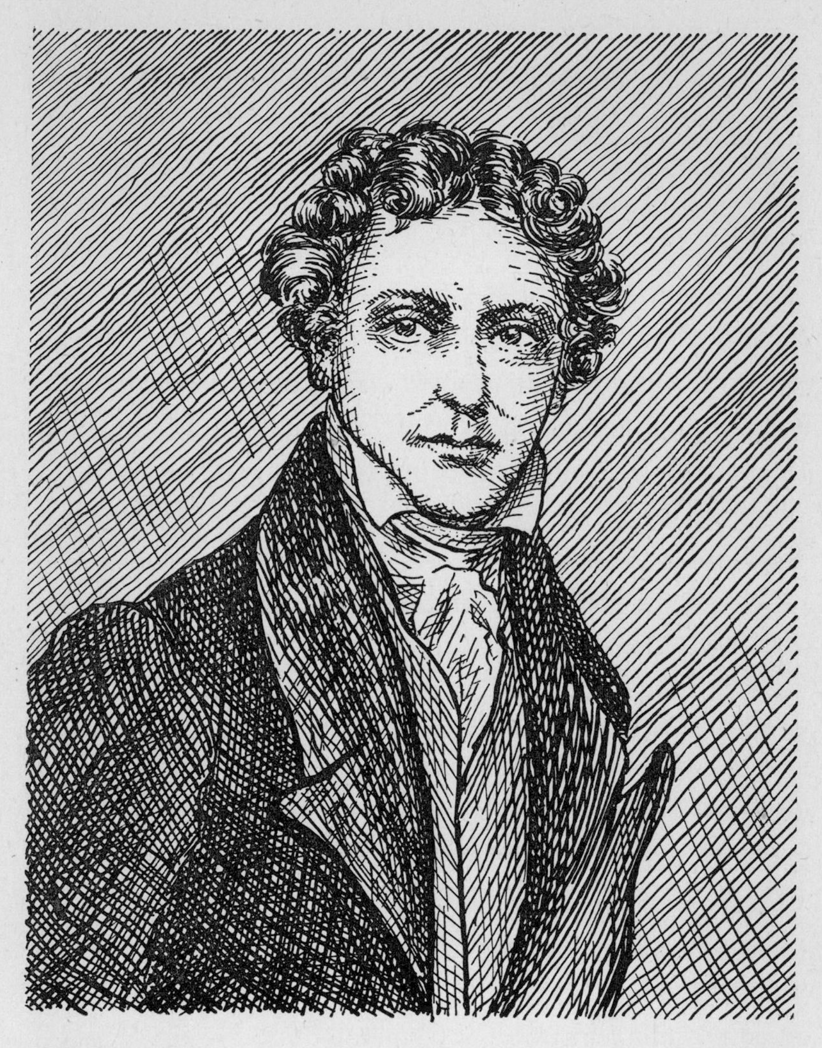

Michael Faraday (1791-1867), whose discovery of induction made possible the development of new therapeutic current applications. The faradic current is named in his honor

III
CONTRACTILE EFFECTS

THE PHYSICAL PROCESSES OF LIFE are dependent upon muscular, sensory, and nutritional *activity*. Currents of electricity applied to the body for their ability to stimulate activity of the nerves and other tissues of the body have an important place among physical therapy procedures. A properly constructed contractile current generator covers a wide field of usefulness, and an attempt will be made in the following pages to show why it is capable of supplying a type of stimulation to the body obtainable from no other method.

The definition of contractile current as used here includes electrical current of any type which may be used safely on the body and is capable of producing contraction of muscle tissue. To workers in the field of electrotherapy who are already familiar with low voltage generators and their applications in therapy, this definition will bring to mind a variety of instruments generating an even greater variety of currents, known by such terms as sine wave, rapid sinusoidal, surging sine, pure sinusoidal, faradism, pulsating direct, slow sine, and many others. In order to avoid possible confusion of terminology the reader is asked to try to judge whatever type of current may be under discussion solely from its immediate physiologic effect on human tissue, without regard to names that have been applied to it in the past.

The purpose of utilizing electrical muscle stimulation

should be to produce contractions which simulate normal voluntary muscular contractions if possible.

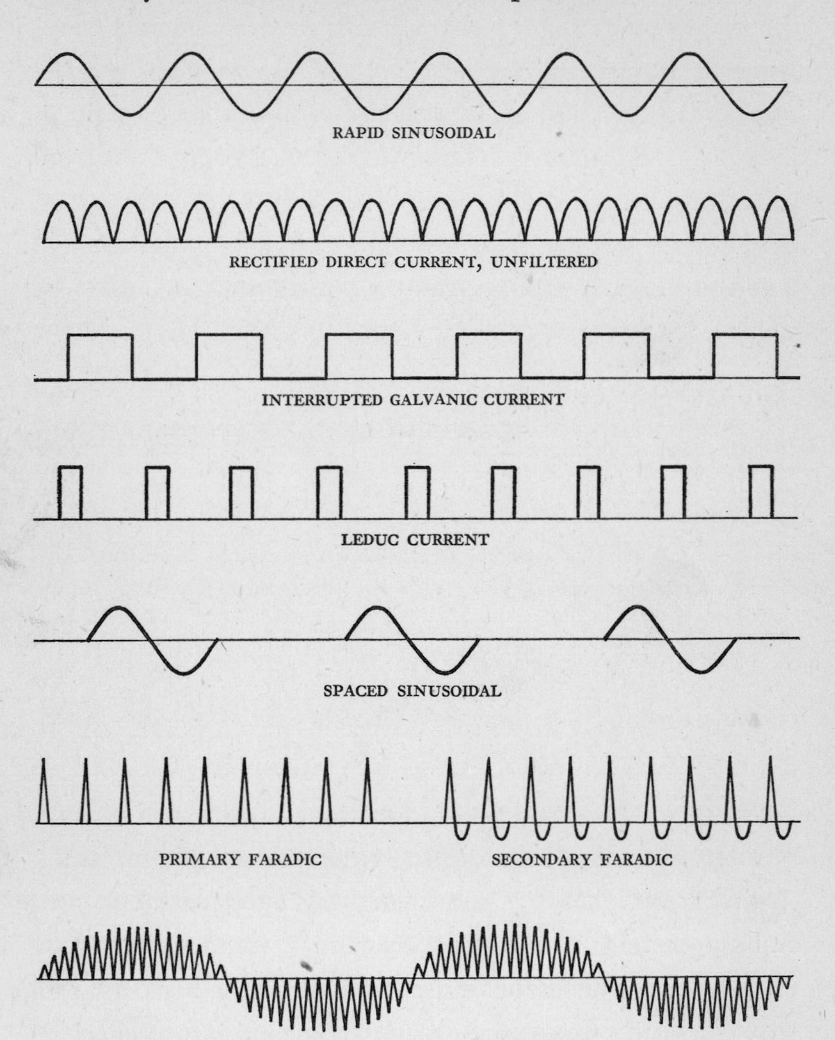

A few of the many types of electric current capable of producing muscular contractions

CONTRACTILE CURRENT CHARACTERISTICS. The one outstanding physical characteristic of a *contractile* current is the *rapid rate of change* in amplitude of the individual electrical pulses that make up the current. To be effective, the rate of change must occur within certain limits of time. It must exceed a minimum rate, the impulse going from zero to maximum in a small fraction of a second. It will be evident, therefore, that if a current is changing in intensity at a rate sufficiently rapid to cause a contraction, it must soon reverse its direction, or momentarily cease, otherwise the

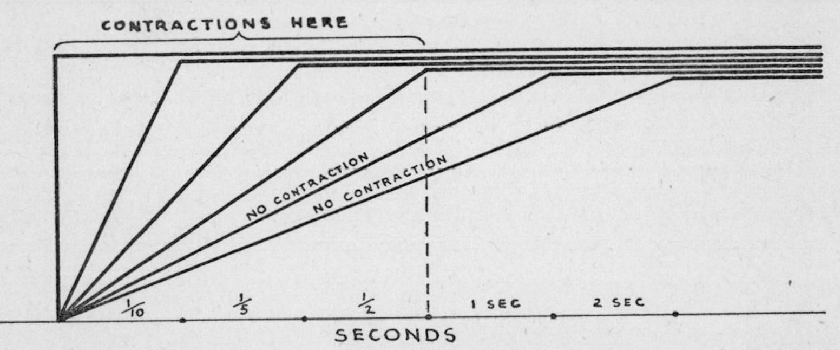

Graph illustrating the necessity for rapid rate of current change in order to produce contractions

intensity of the current would become unbearably large. It must go through certain rapid cyclic changes in intensity.

RAPID SINUSOIDAL. Much stress has been placed on contractile currents of the rapid sinusoidal type, or alternating current as supplied for household use. In spite of the fact that the need for currents of the "true sine" form has been stressed repeatedly, there is no physiological indication whatever for the necessity or advisability of employing this type of current. Electrical currents normally generated in the motor nerves of the body and delivered to the muscles, resulting in muscular contraction, *are not sinusoidal in form.* As a matter of fact, they resemble repetitive bursts of a sequence of pulses, spaced well apart, the individual impulse being similar to the discharge of an electrical condenser.

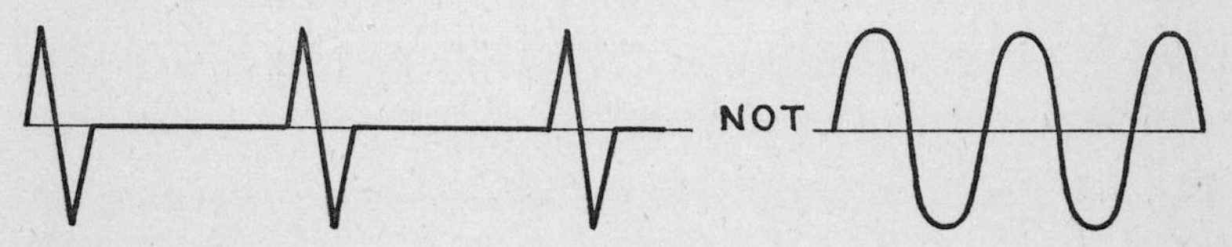

Normal nerve currents consist of spaced impulses, are not sinusoidal in form

PURE SINUSOIDAL. Sinusoidal currents when alternating at a sufficiently rapid rate will cause nerve stimulation and muscular contraction, as will currents of many other types. However, improvement in the application of contractile current therapy may come from accurate observations of normal nerve currents. These currents can be duplicated, in principle at least, so that stimulation from artificial currents will resemble more closely normal muscular activity.

THERAPEUTIC VALUE OF CONTRACTILE CURRENTS. Before going further into the question of what constitutes an ideal contractile current, it might be well first to point out some of the fundamental reasons why contractile currents are of therapeutic value.

PROBLEM OF THERAPY. Muscles have the following characteristics: (1) irritability—the ability to respond to a stimulus, (2) contractility—the ability to shorten when stimulated, (3) extensibility—the ability to regain normal status after being contracted.

One of the greatest problems of therapy is to maintain at least in part the irritability, contractility, and nutrition of muscles which have been immobilized or damaged or which have an impaired nerve supply. A muscle that has been subject to disuse is unable to perform its natural function of contraction, and there is a tendency for it to revert to connective tissue type. Until the opportunity for normal use is restored electrical stimulation helps to preserve at least part of the functional properties of a muscle by causing movements similar to normal muscular activity.

ELECTRIC MASSAGE. The stimulating effects are multiple. Not only does "electric massage" produce all the benefits of physical massage, with its increased drainage of lymph, and general increased circulation, but there is also a direct stimulation to activity in the nerves supplying the area under treatment. The beneficial effect of electrical stimulation on denervated muscle is more pronounced than the effect of manual massage.

VOLUNTARY EXERCISE. Voluntary movement is a most desirable form of activity, and perhaps artificially stimulated activity cannot have exactly the same physiological value. Yet there are many conditions in which natural function is lost or diminished, and it is in the treatment of such conditions that artificial electrical stimulation can be beneficial. Volitional effort on the part of the patient is encouraged, in addition to the usual beneficial nutritional changes resulting from muscle action.

The physical and chemical phenomena connected with normal muscular work are reproduced by electrically stimulated muscular exercise. All the tissues in the neighborhood are benefited by the increased activity, produced by muscle movements, in the blood and lymph. Muscle action also lessens the formation of adhesions, which are a frequent cause of long-standing disability after even minor injuries.

NERVE STIMULATION. The stimulating effects of currents designed for their contractile properties are not limited to muscle contraction. Laboratory experiments with nerve segments have shown that nervous activity may be excited by the same electrical impulses. Some of the effects of increased activity in nerve tissue are: (1) an increase of heat production, (2) an increase in metabolism, and (3) alteration of excitability. The latter effect is of extreme importance. In cases of lessened irritability through degeneration, electrical stimulation tends to increase the nerve irritability. When nerves are in a state of greater irritability than normal (neuritis), electrical stimulation of the nerve tends to lessen the irritability. These apparently contradictory effects have long been observed.

In summary, the principal therapeutic uses of contractile currents of low voltage are: (1) the production of muscular contractions in weak and paralyzed muscles, (2) the restoration of function impaired through injury and muscle weakness, (3) muscle exercise for improvement of muscle tone, for improvement of circulation, and for postural improvement, and (4) nerve stimulation.

RESTORATION OF MUSCLE TONE. It is interesting to note that restoration of muscle tone, the essential factor in producing recovery of deficient muscle function, is brought about by the contractions themselves, and not by the electricity per se. The general effects of electricity are relatively unimportant, although, for instance, there might be a slight heat effect. It is not merely a question of giving a dose of electricity, or of passing the current through the muscles (as is the case when treating with galvanism). Volitional movement (self-excitation) is necessary for improvement. Work must actually be done by the muscles. Contractions induced by correctly patterned electrical currents simulate very closely normal physiological contractions. The stimulation to activity must come from within the muscle, either from volitional movement, or from externally applied electrical impulses. Obviously volitional movements are not possible in paralysis. Passive exercise and massage often will not provide the necessary impetus to influence regeneration of wasted muscles.

JOINT CONDITIONS. Contractile current therapy is of particular importance in the repair of joint injuries, for it is necessary to maintain the muscles operating the joint in a high state of efficiency. It is possible that the muscles may be in such a condition of atrophy following the otherwise complete recovery of a joint, even after what might be described as minor injuries, that no amount of volitional exercise alone will restore them to full activity. Such muscles, if the nerve supply is intact, when correctly stimulated with contractile electrical currents, will show growth of muscle fibres at a far greater rate and of far greater efficiency than would be possible by exercise alone. At the right moment volitional exercise can be called on to increase muscle bulk.

In any inflamed joint there is always the history of early loss of tone of the muscles followed rapidly by wasting of the muscle fibres. It is during this early stage that electrical stimulation applied to the muscles is the most effective aid to their natural repair, and to the repair of other damaged tissues. No damaged joint can be considered to have recovered completely until the tone and contractility of its muscles have been restored to normal.

Muscles are never atonic in health. The part that muscle action plays in the efficiency of the circulatory system is of such importance that serious interference with local and general metabolism may follow the loss or diminution of muscle action from any cause.

EARLY USE IN INJURIES. The therapeutic effects obtainable from the employment of correctly designed and correctly applied contractile currents have been greatly increased by the methods introduced and developed by several European investigators and clinicians, notably Profs. Leduc, Lapicque, Bourguignon, and Sir Morton Smart. It has been shown that electrical stimulation designed to restore muscle tone and prevent atrophy after injury is based on sound physiology and should be carried out as soon as possible.

EFFECT OF MUSCLE MOTION. Dr. Smart has shown that stiffness so common after strains and sprains passes off soon after initial voluntary movements have occurred, and immediately after electrically produced muscular contractions. *Movement*, not rest, is the basis of restoration of function.

Necessary stimulation can be achieved in two ways: (1) by voluntary movement, which in the early stage is not always possible, and (2) by correct application of the right kind of contractile current. Expertly done, this can be applied with perfect safety in all kinds of injured joints, even the most painful.

VALUE OF ELECTRICAL METHOD. The method of electrical stimulation produces painless alternate contractions and relaxations of muscles and so reproduces the beneficial physiochemical changes resulting from muscular activity. Muscle tone is restored, adhesions are prevented, and muscle wasting is lessened. Above all, the blood and lymph supply to the damaged and surrounding parts is stimulated, and thus the rate of repair is increased.

RAPIDITY OF RECOVERY. It should be noted that a definite point of wasting and atonicity may follow injury, and when this is reached no amount of passive or voluntary exercise will cause complete redevelopment. However, the response to contractile current stimulation terminates in rapid and complete recovery, provided the nerve path is intact.

CYCLE OF CONTRACTION. Muscular contraction means not only a simple contraction of muscle fibre, but the complete sequence from the stimulus, which starts the action, to its cessation. It includes the contraction of the principal muscle or group, with shortening and broadening, the inhibition, relaxation, and elongation of the opposing muscles, and the subsequent relaxation of the contracting muscles until a condition of equilibrium is reached between the opposing groups of muscles.

STIMULATION OF INVOLUNTARY MUSCLES. Contractions are produced in voluntary muscles the instant a sufficiently strong impulse is applied. This contraction continues as long as repetitive stimuli are applied in quick succession, and relaxed quickly the instant the stimulating current is removed. When, however, the stomach, the esophagus, the intestines, and other parts which are composed of involuntary muscle fibre are subject to a contractile current, the resulting movements are slightly delayed in starting, and the contractions are a slow, worm-like movement. Moreover, contraction continues a short time after the stimulating current has ceased to flow. Partially degenerated skeletal muscles react to stimulation in a manner similar to that of the involuntary muscles.

NECESSITY FOR SPECIAL CURRENTS. The fact that involuntary muscle can be contracted by electrical stimulation is not questioned. Whether externally applied currents can effectively contract the intestines, or the muscular layers of the stomach, for example, is a question upon which there is some disagreement. It is in stimulation of involuntary muscle that special currents are required, developed on the basis of new knowledge of the functioning of this type of tissue. Some of the experimental failures to accomplish the attempted stimulation of involuntary muscle by practical therapeutic procedures may be due to the fact that currents of a correct pattern were not available.

Involuntary muscles which have been stimulated by direct application (surgical) are those of the stomach, the intestines, the spleen, the bladder, the uterus, the gall bladder, the esophagus, and the smaller arteries. Therefore it is reasonable to suppose that some of these tissues can be stimulated by externally applied currents, *provided* the patient can tolerate sufficient intensity of the current without excessive pain, and without painful tetany of the skeletal muscles adjacent to the electrodes.

CURRENTS FOR INVOLUNTARY MUSCLE STIMULATION. Some of the factors which should characterize a current to be used for stimulation of involuntary muscle, and also for partially degenerated skeletal muscle, are as follows:

1. Absence of surface sting and sensation of burning, contributing factors being: (1) excessively large amount of current necessary to elicit a contraction, (2) excessively high frequency, and (3) electrodes which do not distribute the current evenly over the surface of the skin.

2. Absence of tetanic type contractions. Tetany may be produced by the summation effect of the individual muscle twitches resulting from each impulse that makes up the current. Currents of excessively high frequency produce tetanic-type contractions. The rate of normal innervation of the motor units of the body is anywhere from approximately five to ten per second in slightly contracted muscles to as high as fifty per second in strongly contracted muscles. (The rate of innervation of involuntary muscles is somewhat less.) Even in extreme tetany the rate seldom rises as high as 100 per second. It is reasonable to suppose that frequencies higher than these normal rates should not

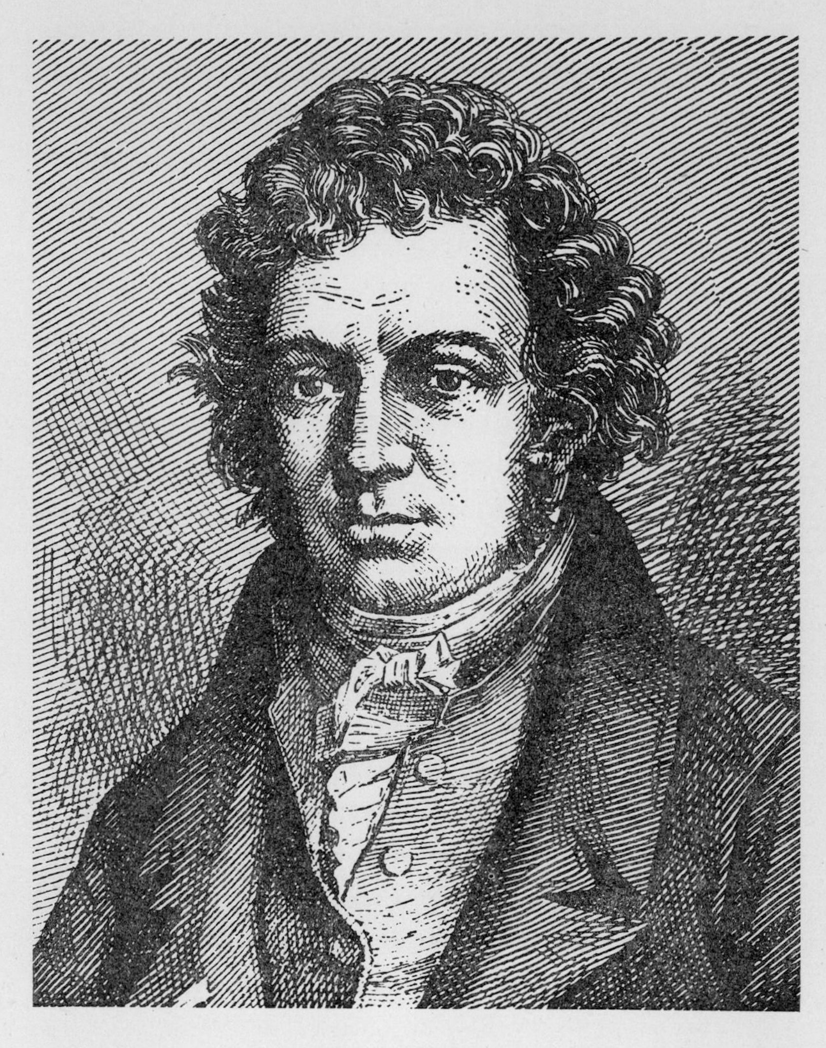

Andre Marie Ampere (1775-1836), French physicist after whom the unit of electric current density, the ampere, is named

be used, since contractions resulting from the higher frequency currents elicit only tetanic-type contractions which are often painful. Many of the contractile currents supplied in standard apparatus have frequencies of several hundred cycles per second. Such currents are not correctly designed for stimulation of involuntary muscle, or denervated skeletal muscle.

3. Deep-seated contractions. The production of deep-seated muscular contractions depends on the use of currents of relatively low frequency (less than fifty per second), in order to prevent tetany of skeletal muscles close to the electrodes, and to utilize the additional activation that may be produced through stimulation of the spinal nerve centers.

4. No residual chemical effect. This is not a *necessary* quality; in fact, some authorities prefer the combination effects of a polarized current, as is produced by the *superimposed* current. When polarized contractile currents are employed in treatments of more than a few minutes' duration it is possible that excessive chemical effects may be produced, resulting in irritation of the skin. Some contractile current generators produce only polarized currents.

5. The current should not produce nerve fatigue or nervous exhaustion. Such effects, resulting in general nervous irritability, may result from prolonged treatment application of currents of excessively high frequency. In order to impart a feeling of "smoothness" to the stimulation resulting from a contractile current application, the frequency of the current is sometimes increased until the current is on the threshold of losing its contractile power entirely.

Roughly, this is between 2,000 and 3,000 cycles per second. Such a current may induce nerve fatigue, possibly of value in the treatment of some conditions, *but which defeats one of the objectives of deep-seated contractile stimulation*—namely, *nerve stimulation.*

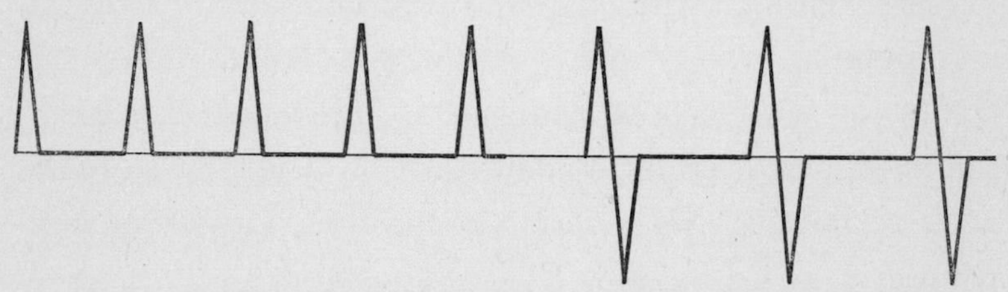

Monophasic and diphasic spaced impulses

THE IDEAL CONTRACTILE CURRENT. What is the best contractile current? Opinions differ widely. Some authorities insist that contractile currents be "true sinusoidal" in form. Others recommend the interrupted galvanic current, or the slowly surging galvanic current with alternating polarity. A few still adhere to the opinion that the "Morton wave" static is of greatest value. Perhaps some of this diversity of opinion is due to the fact that each type of current will work in certain conditions, will not work in others. Also, apparatus has not been available that permits adjustment of the type of stimulus in accordance with the changing irritability encountered in various degrees of degeneration. In a few cases it is possible that investigators have attempted to adjust their concept of electrophysiology to fit the currents to which they had been limited in their work. An examination of the nature of action currents present in bodily nerves during muscular activity may suggest the currents that will best meet the requirements listed above.

ACTION UNIT. According to Erlanger and Gasser, the action unit of a motor impulse resembles the wave form of the discharge of a condenser through resistance. It is a spike impulse, with fixed timing as to duration and intensity. It is sometimes monophasic, sometimes diphasic. In the low frequency sequences of mild activity it is nonpolarized. In the higher frequencies, which result in vigorous muscular activity, there is a polarization effect, which probably contributes to rapid fatigue.

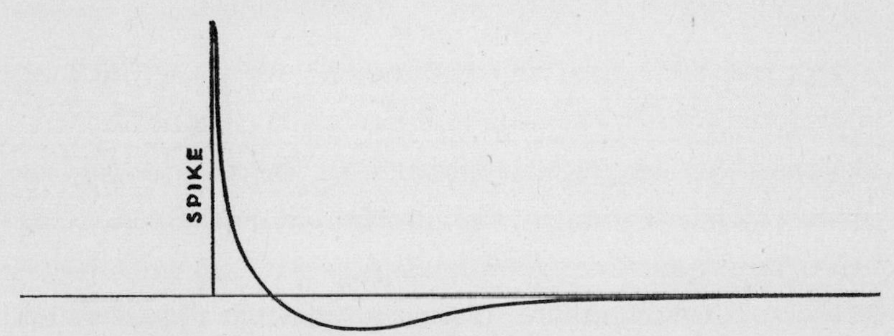

Theoretical "action unit" of motor nerve current

From the above observations, our "ideal" contractile current should be designed with the following factors in mind: (1) an "action unit" of such amplitude and duration that it will cause contractile stimulation to normal and partially degenerated muscle alike, without excessive sensation of pain; (2) a sequence of such potentials, or spikes, the frequency of which can be varied in order to obtain variable contractile effects all the way from extreme tetanic response of the stimulated muscle, on the one hand, to the spaced individual contractile impulses characterized by the sharp momentary muscle twitch from the "static" discharge on the other. Somewhere in this wide range of frequency variation should be found the current that is best suited to the type of muscle to be stimulated. For stimulation of muscles with intact nerve supply it appears possible

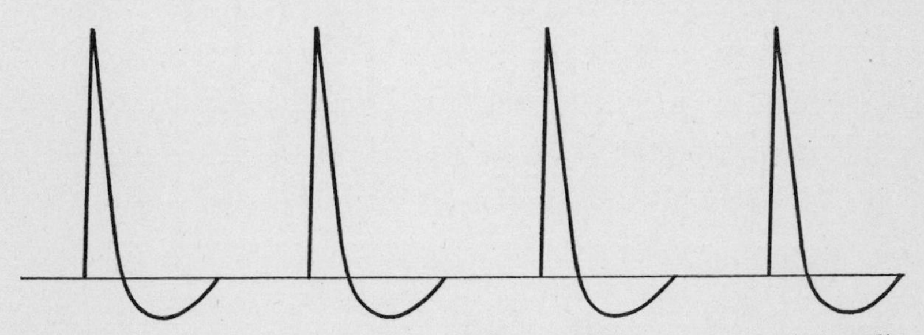

Artificial stimulating current, similar in form to spaced faradic current, patterned after normal action currents

that the ideal current is a sequence of short "spiked" impulses with instantaneous rise, of relatively short duration, and with a frequency of fifty or sixty per second. For degenerated muscles and muscles with impaired nerve supply the individual impulses should perhaps be longer, with either gradual or instantaneous rise, and of a somewhat lower frequency. Where there is considerable degeneration of muscle it may be necessary to utilize the filtered direct (galvanic) current, interruptedly, or in rhythmic surges, in order to obtain "action units" of sufficient duration to produce contractions. The chief requirement of a current when used for the treatment of denervated muscle is that it will produce a *contraction* of the muscle, and the effectiveness of any contractile current must be judged by that ability. For a muscle with some of its fibres denervated and other fibres with the nerve supply intact, care must be taken to use a current that will stimulate the denervated fibres.

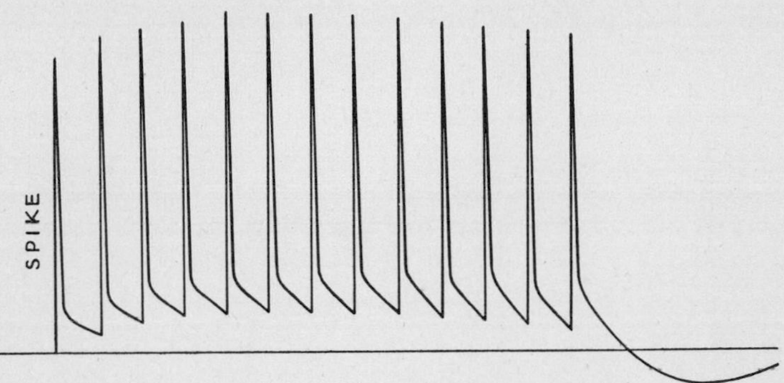

Graph of action current producing a tetanus

As previously mentioned, motor nerve currents are like bursts of machine-gun bullets, with varying frequency of discharge, but with fairly constant amplitude and duration. They do not in any way resemble "rapid sinusoidal" currents. No matter what the frequency of the discharge of a motor nerve might be there is a refractory or rest period after each impulse that is longer in duration than the actual spike impulse. The spikes, for example, may be of only 1/1000th of a second duration each, but they are spaced well apart so that only 5 or 10 or 25 or 40 per second are supplied, the rate varying with the degree of muscular contraction being elicited. The interval of spacing is much longer than the motor part of the action unit. An ideal instrument with which to carry on research work would be one in which both the shape and duration of the impulse, and the frequency, could be controlled.

TYPES OF MUSCULAR CONTRACTIONS. Experiments with

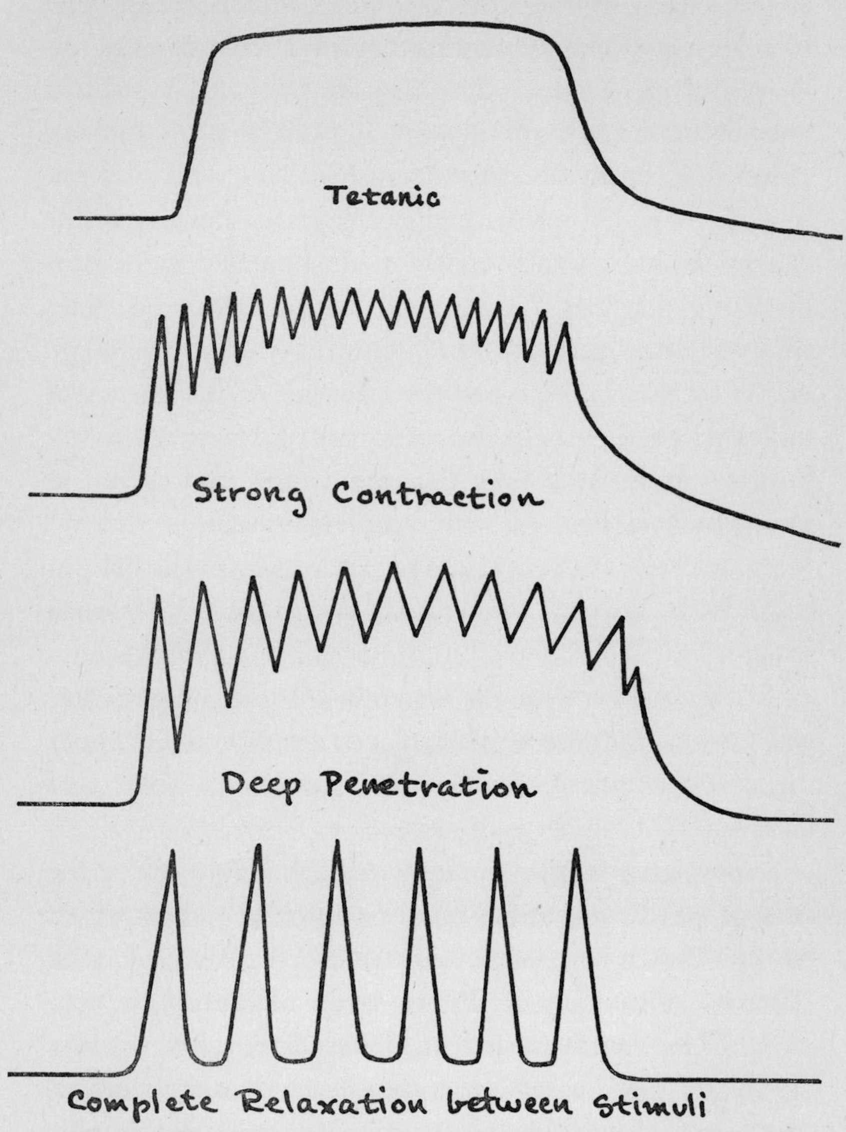

1. *Above 100 per sec.* 2. *30-60 per sec.* 3. *10-30 per sec.* 4. *1-5 per sec.*

Types of muscular contractions produced by currents of various frequencies

a wide variety of frequencies, ranging from one per second to as high as several thousand per second, show that the following types of contractions may be produced in muscles with intact nerve supply by varying the frequency of impulse-type contractile currents:

1. *Tetanic.* All of the higher frequency ranges capable of stimulating muscular contractions dominate in the production of tetanic contractions in the muscles immediately adjacent to the electrodes, and in the muscles innervated by nerves so stimulated, when the intensity of the current is increased to slightly above threshold. This effect is not lessened appreciably until the frequencies are lowered to somewhat less than one hundred per second.

2. *Smooth contractive.* As the frequency of the current is gradually lowered to about the range found in normal innervation of heavy volitional muscular activity (about 45 per second) the muscle response is brisk and effective, and greater intensity of current can be tolerated without the extreme tetany produced by the higher frequency currents.

3. *Deep penetrative.* By lowering the frequency of the current still further, to as low as 15 per second, at which rate the muscles are permitted to relax slightly after each "twitch," the effect of deeper stimulation may be produced. The contractile effect is cumulative, but without the tetany that characterizes the muscular stimulation of the higher-frequency currents. The response to each individual "action impulse" can be felt as a distinct contraction, and the intensity of current that can be tolerated

comfortably is far above threshold intensity. Since the surface muscles can tolerate this increased intensity, the deeper seated muscles, both voluntary and involuntary, have a better chance to be reached with threshold-intensity stimuli, and thus they too may be stimulated. Of course the quality of electrical penetration has not been changed; what has been affected is the patient's tolerance to greatly increased intensities of current.

Furthermore, the lower frequency currents come closer to the normal rates of innervation of the deep-seated involuntary muscles, which probably have a maximum rate of innervation not higher than five to fifteen per second, possibly less. These low frequency "intermittent" currents, as they are sometimes called, are sometimes effective where other currents have failed to produce results.

4. *Decongestive*. "Static" currents of the Morton wave type are sharply spiked impulsed spaced well apart, with a frequency of approximately one to three per second. These currents produce sharp muscular contractions, with deep penetrative action, without pain. For many years users of static apparatus have extolled the virtues of condenser discharge currents. Currents with the same physiological effects, but without the objectional features of the frictional apparatus used to generate them, are now available in modern electronic apparatus. Static currents are particularly useful for their decongestive effects in the treatment of pelvic inflammation, sprains, gall bladder, and prostate conditions. Static currents are also very effective in painless electrodiagnostic procedures.

SURGING CURRENTS. Regardless of the nature of the basic currents employed for the purpose of eliciting muscular contractions, it is generally considered necessary to apply them in rhythmic on-and-off intervals, or with periodic surges of power. Muscular relaxation must be provided as well as muscular contraction, in order to make use

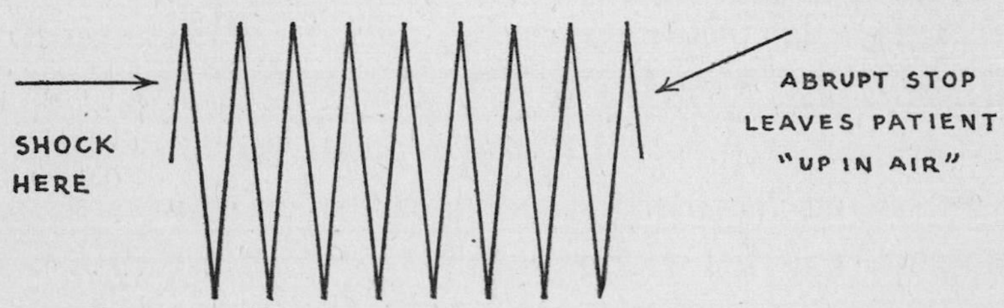

Diagram showing effects of interrupted currents with instantaneous "make" and "break"

of the full stimulating power of the current. This is accomplished by some mechanical or electronic means of producing rhythmic modulations of current intensity, varying slowly from zero to maximum, and back to zero. These surges may be varied anywhere from a few per minute, to as many as one or more per second. A simple snapping of the current on and off with a switch will produce unpleasant shocks to the patient, so the increase and decrease of current intensity should be gradual, regardless of the surge speed employed.

SURGE TIMING. It is advisable to give consideration to the type of contraction desired, and so the question of determining the speed of the rhythmic contraction cycles to be used is of some importance. Comparatively slow rates of surge, 12 to 18 per minute, are generally employed for stimulation of involuntary muscles and for muscles that show considerable degeneration. Faster rates of surge, 20 to 60 per minute, are employed for voluntary muscle stimulation where the nerve path is intact. A pronounced "dwell" is important, especially when stimulating involuntary muscles, because of the longer time the muscle takes to

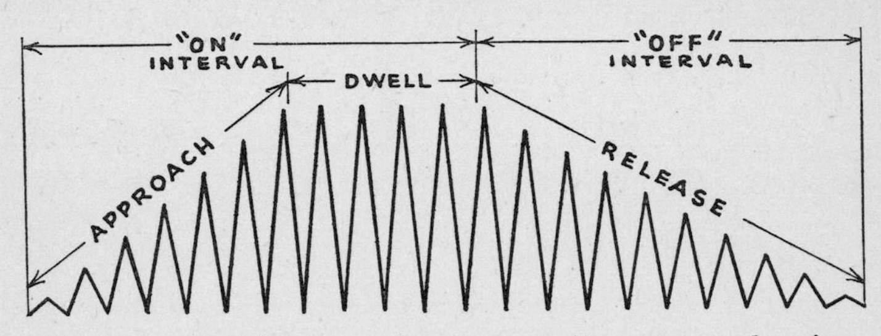

Analysis of cycle of surging contractile current, showing graduated "approach" and "release"

respond to the stimulus. With some of the newer contractile current instruments the flexibility of the electronic controls permits a wide variety of surge timing, where the shape of the surge wave can be set in any way desired. Care should be taken not to confuse the basic current frequency (cycles per *second*) with the timing of the surge rhythm (surges per *minute*).

In setting the surge frequency (surges per minute) the normal contraction rate of the parts to be treated should be considered. If the muscles of the arms healthfully exercise or contact at from 20 to 40 times per minute, the respiratory muscles at from 18 to 22 times per minute, involuntary at a slower rate than voluntary, and so on for different fuctions of the body, it may not be good therapy to apply currents with contraction rates that differ too greatly from the normal rates.

ELECTRODES. Contractile current electrodes are usually identical with the ones used for galvanism, except that in the treatment of local areas smaller electrodes often may be used. There is practically no danger of local burn due to excessive current, and therefore bare metal electrodes may sometimes be used where there is good contact with moist

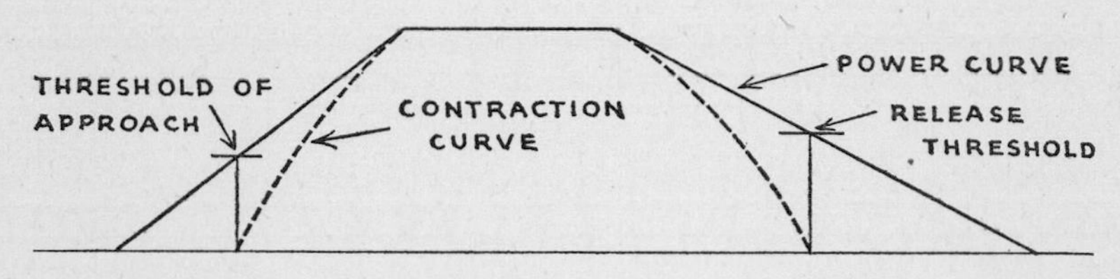

Contraction curve does not coincide with power curve

skin surface. When electrodes of unequal size are used the contractile effect may be stronger at the smaller electrode, but this is not always the case since the location of the nerve centers and motor points largely determines the sensitivity. Usually the smaller electrode is termed the active, although in most applications the two electrodes are of equal size. Two or more electrodes may be connected in parallel on each side of the circuit if it is necessary to cover a greater area than the largest single electrode available.

PLACEMENT OF ELECTRODES. Careful study of the placement of active and indifferent electrodes should be made. Indifferent electrodes should be placed at areas of least motor sensitivity, such as the chest or back. When electrodes of approximately the same size are used, both are considered active. Active electrodes should be placed over motor areas, or spinal nerve centers. In glandular, visceral, and other treatments of deep-seated conditions, one electrode should be placed over the area to be treated, and the other electrode over the center of spinal innervation of the part or region. Or stimulation may be made through the spinal nerve centers only, by placing both electrodes adjacent to the spinal center, one on each side of the spine, about two inches apart.

DOSAGE. In all contractile current treatments the most reliable guide to the intensity of current to be used is the degree of muscular contraction. A milliammeter may be used with the higher frequency currents as a guide to repeating a treatment, but the initial guide to maximum intensity is the patient's reaction. When treating a patient for the first time watch for "psychological contractions," which may be due to nervousness and are not a correct indication of current intensity.

FREQUENCY OF TREATMENT. The frequency with which the treatments can be given may be determined by the reaction of the patient. It is generally advisable to treat every day, or at least every other day. The reaction to watch for is a mild soreness of the muscle, the day following treatment. As the strength of the muscles increases the duration and intensity of the treatment can gradually be increased.

TYPES OF ELECTRODE APPLICATIONS. Three general types of electrode applications are employed for contractile current stimulation:

1. *Motor point stimulation.* By this method the current strength is concentrated at the motor point of the muscle

to be treated. A somewhat larger indifferent electrode is used so that there will be no stimulation except at the motor point. A modification of this technic is called the method of longitudinal excitation. Two equal-size small electrodes are used, one at each end of the muscle.

The patient should be placed in a comfortable position, where the parts to be treated are warm and relaxed. A preliminary warming with infra-red or other heat generator is sometimes advisable, especially when the skin is dry. The indifferent electrode is placed on any convenient part of the body where there is little sensitivity to the current. The active electrode should be a ball or disc, not over 1 to 1½ inches in diameter, possibly smaller for some muscles of the face. It should be covered with felt, gauze, or chamois, and it should be kept well-moistened. A contractile current, surging at a fairly rapid rate (45 to 60 per minute) should be used for stimulating muscles with intact nerve supply; a lower frequency (10 to 15 per second) contractile current, with a slower rate of surge (12 to 20 per minute) for muscles that show considerable degeneration. The intensity should be sufficient to produce mild contraction. Each muscle should be treated separately.

The signs of overstimulation are lessened speed of contraction, and stiffness and pain several hours after treatment. At the first sign of fatigue during treatment the electrode should be shifted to another motor point, or the treatment terminated.

2. *Group stimulation of muscles.* This technic takes advantage of the fact that all muscles supplied by a nerve can

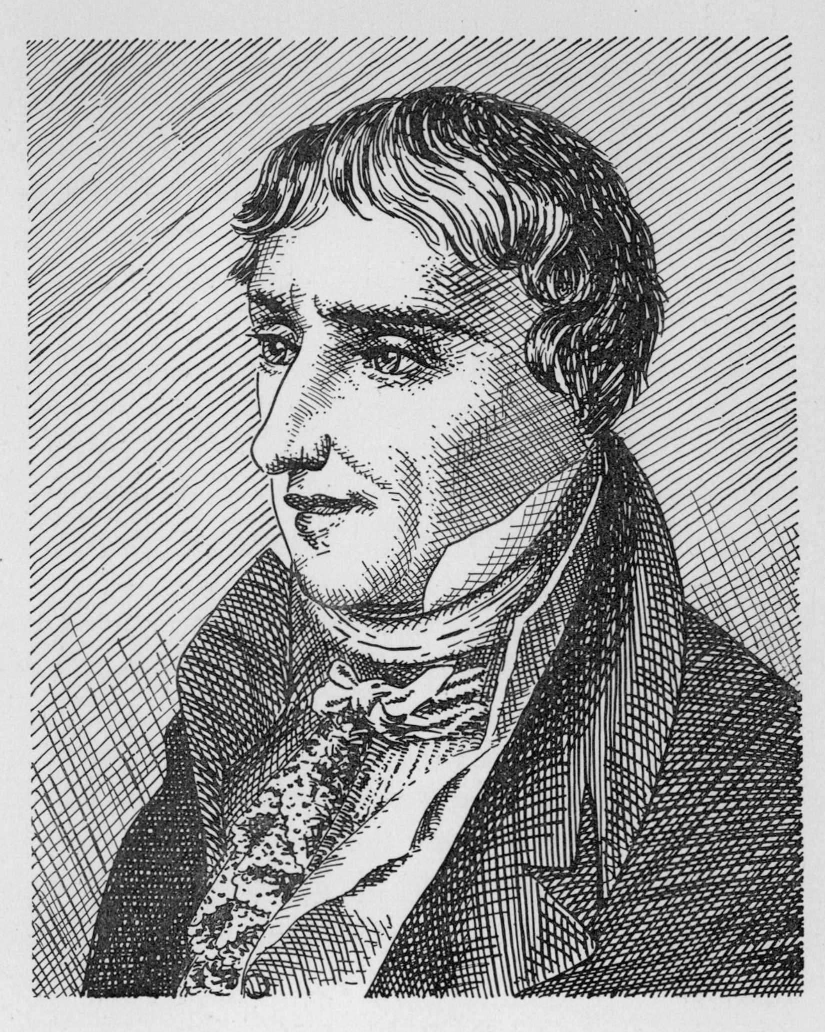

Alessandro Volta (1745-1827), a celebrated pioneer of electrical science, after whom the volt, the unit of electrical pressure, is named

be stimulated at one time through the nerve. The electrodes, generally of medium or large size, may be applied to each end of an extremity, or longitudinally, over the nerve path. General technic and rules are about the same as with individual motor-point stimulation. In after-treatment of fractures, or in treatment for adhesions of the extremities following operations for infections, the group stimulation method may be effectively employed.

3. *Stimulation through the spinal nerve centers.* Two medium-size electrodes (about 3″ x 3″) may be placed on each side of the spine, about two inches apart, adjacent to the spinal area from which the nerves to the area to be treated emerge. For example, the viscera may be stimulated by placing two equal-size electrodes over the 7th and 8th dorsal area of the spine, one electrode on each side. Or a modification of the group stimulation method may be used by placing one electrode over the area to be stimulated, and the other electrode over the area of spinal innervation of the part. In the abdominal treatment outlined above, one large electrode is used over the abdominal area, and one smaller electrode is used over the 7th and 8th dorsal region of the spine. In either case a comparatively low frequency deep-penetrative contractile current should be employed. The contractile results will be similar with the use of either technic.

ELECTRIC MASSAGE. The position of massage as a therapeutic agent in both local and systemic application is firmly established. Massage exerts certain physiological effects which can be utilized in a wide variety of conditions. Mul-

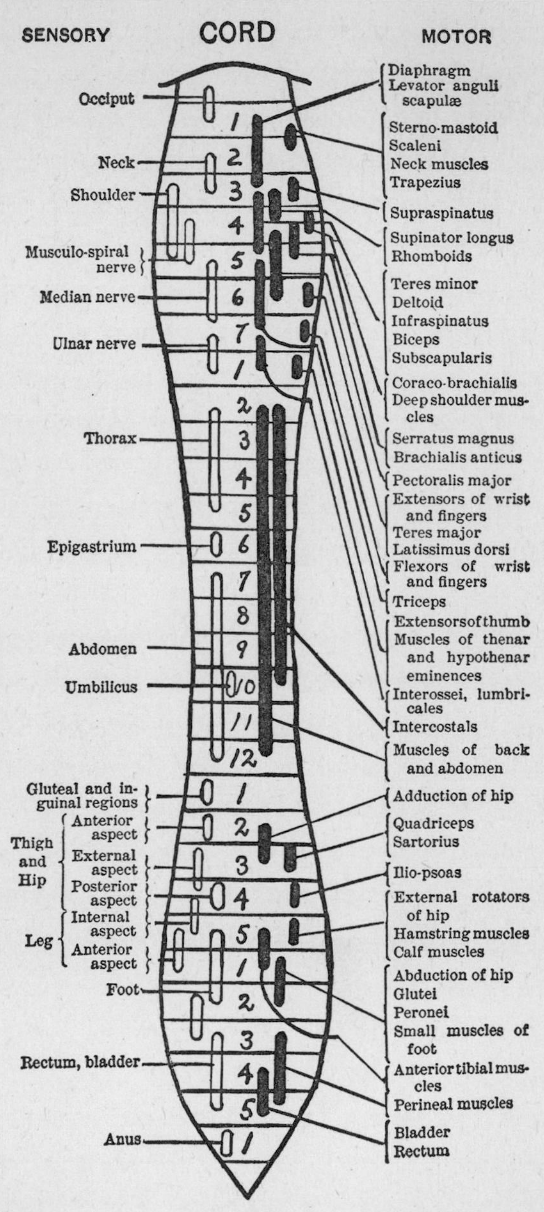

Chart illustrating the importance of correct placement of electrodes for stimulation through the spinal nerve centers

tiple electrical muscular stimulation apparently produces the same type of benefits as manual massage, such as increase of peripheral blood flow and resulting metabolic increment. The flow of lymph is accelerated, and the removal of debris incident to trauma is hastened. The beneficial effects are present, without the hard manual work.

STATIC. The therapeutic effects of the static discharge currents are largely due to the contractile stimulation resulting from the individual spaced discharge impulses. Modern static currents produce the same deep-penetrating decongestive effects as produced with the original static wave generators, without the massive equipment, and without the high-voltage sparks. There is a definite massage effect, without tetany.

DIRECT CURRENT STIMULATION. The use of the galvanic current for the purpose of producing muscular contractions should be limited to denervated muscles where degeneration has progressed to the stage where the muscle fails to respond to the shorter impulses of the contractile current without the current "splashing over" to the adjacent muscles. Muscles with intact nerve supply should be stimulated with short-impulse currents, because less surface irritation is produced.

EXAMPLES OF CONTRACTILE CURRENT APPLICATIONS

PARALYSIS. Most forms of paralysis respond best to individual motor point stimulation, although group stimulation may be used in some instances. The static-type impulses, applied with a motor-point electrode, are valuable in testing the individual contractile power of the muscles, and in making the initial treatments, as contractions can be elicited without tetany or pain. For continued treatment, surging currents of relatively low frequency are recommended, applied to each muscle and each nerve trunk. *Surging direct currents should be employed only where conventional currents fail to produce contractions.*

Any patient with flaccid paresis with possibility of reinnervation should be treated by contractile stimulation, and that treatment must be continued at least until reinnervation has begun. Treatments should not be withheld until the muscles are in a state of advanced degeneration.

In cases where reinnervation cannot be expected the problem is more difficult. In cases of poliomyelitis, in which trophic disturbances are often responsible for many of the patients' symptoms, there seems to be indication for electrical stimulation.

If paretic muscles are constantly stimulated the patients retain to some extent the "sensations of contraction," and it is easier for them to "find the innervation" when active contraction occurs. Both paretic and normal muscles must be induced to contract.

NEURITIS. Several approaches may be made to the problem of treatment of neuritis by electrical stimulation. Prolonged applications (20 to 45 minutes) of faradic-type currents, applied in sub-contractile intensity, are sometimes effective. Other cases respond to surging contractile stimulation. One author has reported as effective the application through the nerve of intense, tetanizing stimulations of rapid sinusoidal currents, nonsurging, of only one to three minutes' duration.

CONSTIPATION. In constipation the response seems to be best to the deep-penetrative stimulation of currents of relatively low frequency, applied in slow surges. Application of the electrodes may be made directly to the abdomen, consecutively over the three flexures. Or the abdominal muscles may be stimulated through the autonomic nervous system by the application of electrodes parallel to the spine, about two inches apart, at the 7th and 8th dorsal area. The intensity of the current should be the greatest that can be tolerated by the patient, and treatments should be given daily. The surge rate should be from 10 to 18 per minute. A minimum of two or three weeks of treatment is usually necessary to show improvement in bowel action.

VISCEROPTOSIS. For the treatment to be effective the viscera must be elevated if prolapsed, and the abdominal muscles must be contracted. This lifting and contracting stimulus can be supplied by the deep-penetrating currents, with slow surge rhythm of anywhere from 10 to 18 surges per minute. One electrode should be placed over the spine, at the 7th and 8th dorsal area, the other electrode on the abdomen just above the umbilicus. Daily treatments should be given, with current strength sufficient to produce strong contractions, and duration sufficient to produce slight muscular soreness a few hours following treatment.

ABDOMINAL ADHESIONS. Deep-penetrative contractile stimulation, combined with heat therapy, has produced favorable results in relieving the pain of abdominal adhesions and in preventing their formation following surgery. Moist pad electrodes on the back and abdomen will conduct sufficient current to produce the desired exercising effects. Daily treatments with slowly surging currents should be given, of sufficient duration to produce muscular fatigue.

UTERINE SUBINVOLUTION. An insulated metal electrode should be used, preferably a cone-shaped electrode that will direct the current through the uterus to the broad ligaments. The indifferent electrode should be placed over the lumbar spine. Use a surge rate of 15 to 20 per minute of low frequency contractile current.

LUMBAGO. Apply static or contractile current through an electrode large enough to cover the acutely painful area. The intensity should be the maximum that can be tolerated, with duration of 15 to 20 minutes, repeated daily.

FLAT FOOT. Stimulate the tibialis anticus by placing a small electrode over the inner side of the knee, just below the inner tuberosity of the tibia, and another electrode at the inner edge of the affected foot. Treat with strong contractions, 30 to 45 per minute, 10 to 15 minutes daily. Bifurcated cords may be used to treat both feet simultaneously.

BRUISES. The short contractile impulses of the static-type currents may be used for their decongestive action. Also, the superimposed current, with sufficient intensity to produce a mild contraction, 30 surges per minute, positive pole to the pathology, makes use of both the chemical and contractile effects of this current.

OBESITY. A modification of the original Bergonie method of simultaneous multiple stimulation is used in many weight-control establishments today. When combined with restricted caloric intake this method is very effective in correcting postural sluggishness and in maintaining general muscle tone. Body measurements may be reduced without corresponding loss of weight in some cases because of the greater density of firm muscle fibre.

Electrodes, as many as 10 or 12 at a time, are so placed that muscular contractions are produced most heavily in the areas to be reduced in size. The loss of weight is progressive and often permanent, and the treatment is based on the theory that proper use of any organ increases its vitality, and also influences the vitality of the entire body. This is brought about by making the muscles of the body contract and relax through electrical stimulation, or "electric massage." "Spot reducing" makes use of this principle, as does the employment of certain of the facial mask treatments.

In general, the technic for obesity consists of attaching electrodes to the fleshy parts of the arms, legs, thighs, and abdomen. Sand bags and elastic bandages are used to keep the electrodes in place. A rapidly surging contractile current is employed, and sometimes the rate of surge is varied for different individuals or for different parts of the body. The sand bags and elastic bandages may also provide resistance for muscular effort. Actual work must be done by the muscles to accomplish the desired result, which is the production of muscular fatigue. The time of such individual treatments may be as long as 40 to 60 minutes.

FRACTURES. The treatment of fractures is largely a soft tissue problem, and contractile stimulation should be administered to the muscles controlling the functioning of the part as soon as possible. In many cases treatment can be started while traction is still being used. The degree of initial contractile effort must be minimal, so there will be no possibility of disturbing the site of the fracture. The formation of adhesions can be lessened and the possibility of atrophy minimized. Individual motor points should be stimulated, with mild intensity.

SPRAINS AND DISLOCATIONS. The condition of adjacent muscles resembles that accompanying fractures, and similar early treatment should be instituted. The static-type impulse is of value in initiating early treatment, for it produces a momentary muscular impulse that relaxes before joint motion results. Nerve trunks and individual motor points both should be stimulated, starting with only threshold intensity.

ELECTRONARCOSIS. "Shock therapy" is a specialized form of electrical stimulation of the central nervous system in which comparatively large intensities of contractile currents of the "rapid sinusoidal" type are employed (as much as 500 ma.). Special instruments are necessary to produce the amount of current needed and to supply accurate dosage control.

IV
THERMAL EFFECTS

THE EMPLOYMENT of currents of electricity for their thermal effects is generally termed diathermy, meaning "heat-through." Other similar terms are short wave diathermy, short wave therapy, ultra short wave therapy, and (more recently) microtherapy, the terminology used depending somewhat on the relative frequency of the currents employed. For the purposes of this discussion the term short wave therapy will be used to describe the popular form of high frequency apparatus now efficiently employed by thousands of physicians and hospitals all over the world.

The object of this discussion is to review some of the data which have a bearing on the satisfactory operation of short wave apparatus so that present or prospective users of short wave equipment may have a better understanding of the theory and application of the therapy. Certain unique characteristics of short wave therapy cannot be ignored if the best possible results are to be obtained from its use. It is important for the technician to know something of the nature of short wave apparatus, how it works, just what may be expected from the therapy, and what the possible dangers from its use are.

Short wave therapy is essentially *thermal therapy*. It may be considered to be a refinement of d'Arsonval's method of high-frequency heating first presented in 1892, although it was not until approximately 1925 or 1926 that the non-

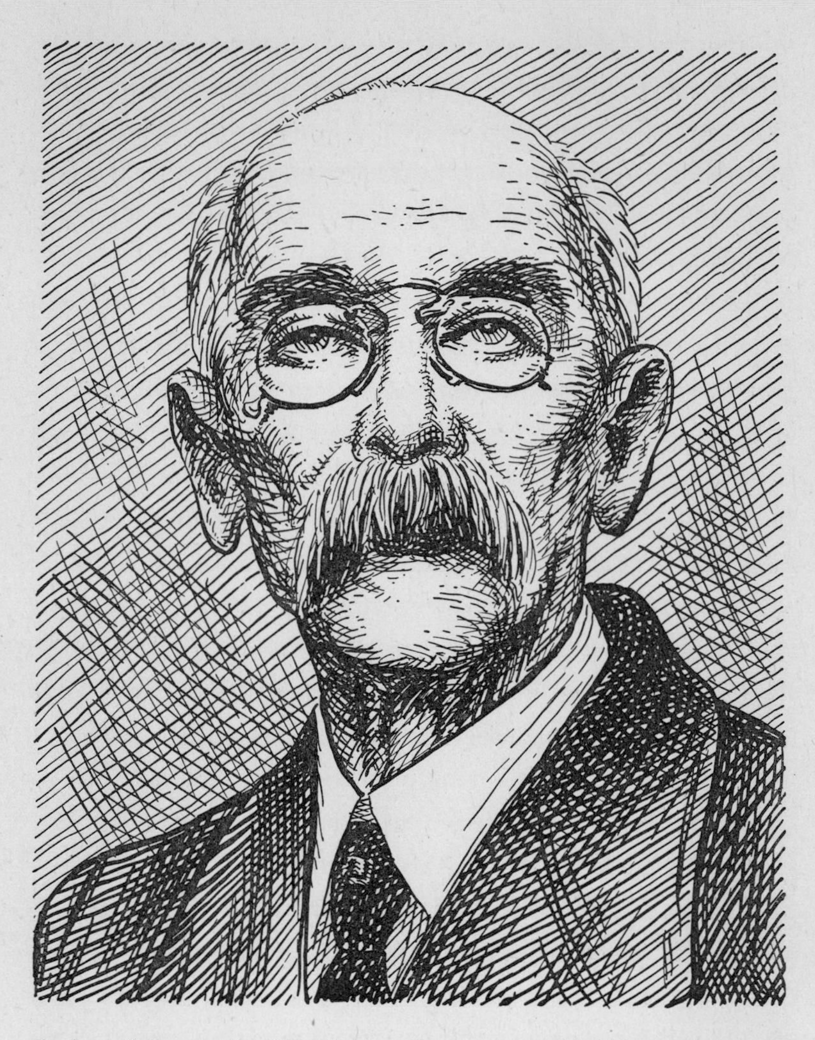

Arsène d'Arsonval, of Paris, in 1891 passed a high frequency current through the human body with no resulting sensation other than heat

contact methods we now use were first investigated. When "short wave" instruments finally were perfected for general use they rapidly displaced the older "spark-gap" instruments. The ease of application of the newer method was probably the deciding factor in making earlier type instruments obsolete.

A short wave diathermy instrument resembles in construction a short wave radio transmitter. The chief difference lies in the fact that the transmitter is designed to radiate energy from antennas as in broadcasting, whereas with the therapy instrument the energy is largely confined between condenser plates, or within or adjacent to an inductive field of a coil.

In operation, a short wave generator might be called an electrical engine for generating currents of rapidly changing polarity. A two-tube generator is similar to a two-cylinder engine, a one-tube instrument similar to a single-cylinder engine. Both a single-cylinder engine and a two-cylinder engine may be equally powerful and efficient. Instead of a heavy rotating flywheel, the short wave "engine" has a tank coil, which is a flywheel of electronic energy just like the flywheel of a steam engine is a reservoir of kinetic mass energy. Each tube (cylinder) consists of a grid (valve) for timing the electrical impulses, and a plate (piston) for receiving and conveying the impulses to the tank coil (flywheel). Or the tank coil could be compared to a pendulum as the electrical charge swings back and forth from end to end of the coil, and the rapidity with which this oscillation takes place determines the frequency, or cycles per second.

To illustrate how this rapidly oscillating electrical energy is transferred to the body to be transformed into heat, let us examine an electrical condenser. A condenser is any arrangement of conductors, usually thin plates, separated by insulating material, the arrangement being capable of holding an electrical charge. In its simplest form it consists of only two conducting plates, with air or other insulating material between them. When an electrical charge is impressed on one plate of a condenser, an equal and *opposite* charge is induced on the other plate. This charge is always on the *surface* of the plate. Essentially, a short wave diathermy consists of an oscillator which is a source of rapidly changing electrical polarity with two condenser plates coupled with the oscillation system. Thus, when one plate has a positive charge the other plate has a negative charge.

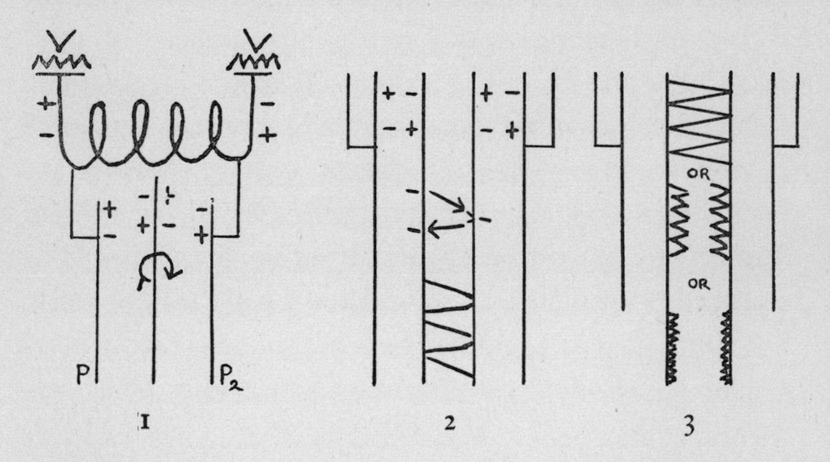

When a reversal of polarity takes place on one plate, a corresponding change takes place on the other plate.

Diagram 1 shows what happens in the oscillating system

when a thin sheet of conductive material (copper) is introduced between the condenser plates. Opposite electrical charges are induced on the surfaces of the copper plate even though it is insulated from the other two plates, and the surface charges of the middle plate will change sides with the changes in polarity of the oscillator plates. Since these charges merely have to travel through the thickness of the plate, from surface to surface, there is little resistance, and practically no energy loss.

If a thick plate of copper is now substituted for the thin center plate, it will be seen that with every change in polarity of the oscillator plates the surface charge has to move from one side to the other. These electrical charges traveling from side to side of the thick center plate constitute an electrical current, the resistance to the flow of which results in energy loss (heat). There is little heating in the copper plate because it is a very good conductor of electricity. If a portion of the body is substituted for the thick copper plate, however, considerable heat will be generated by this oscillatory flow of electric current, because the body has a very much greater resistance to the current flow, and heat will be produced within the tissues. The actual eddy currents created within the body may be small, but with a frequency of many millions per second the heating effects of short wave currents can readily be understood.

Electrically, the short wave oscillator functions as a three-plate condenser system coupled with a master oscillator, and with a portion of the body taking the place of the middle plate. It is the energy *loss* in this high-resistance middle plate that is of importance in short wave therapy. In other words, the heating efficiency of a short wave diathermy is represented by the electrical inefficiency of the middle plate of this three-plate condenser system oscillating in parallel with the short wave generator.

When an inductive coil or treatment drum is used as the applicator instead of the two capacitative plates, the heating effects are similar, except that the heating is due to the resistance within the tissues to the flow of eddy currents inductively set up in the body by the flow of current in the coil. In either case the heat is produced as the result of resistance to the flow of the high frequency eddy currents.

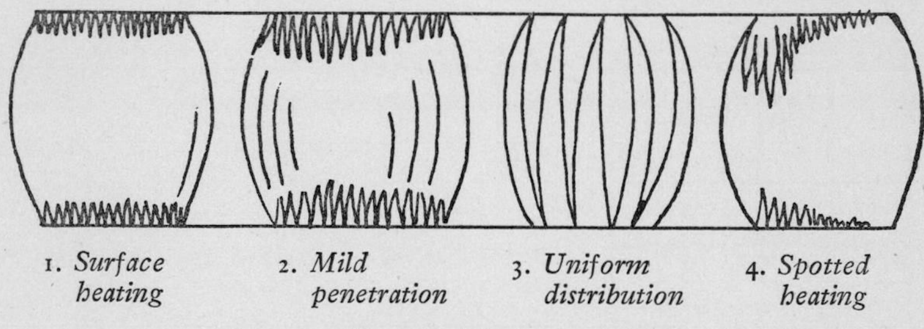

1. *Surface heating* 2. *Mild penetration* 3. *Uniform distribution* 4. *Spotted heating*

Penetration of short wave energy

The real problem of short wave diathermy is the control of the distribution of the heat energy produced. It is incorrect to assume that the energy absorbed by the body from the radiation of a short wave field is uniformly distributed throughout the tissues. Numerous burns have been reported from short wave applications and these would have been impossible if the heating of the tissues had been uniform throughout. With all short wave treatments there is a thermal gradient varying from the hot skin to the less heated deeper tissues. The heating may be fairly uniform, or spotted, or almost entirely on the surface, depending on the design of the equipment and *on factors very largely under the control of the technician.*

In general, for a given amount of surface heating there is a greater amount of penetrative heat with the shorter wave lengths, or greater spacing between the patient and the electrode. For a given wave length greater spacing of electrodes may decrease the total amount of energy applied to the area under treatment, but will increase the proportion of the heat that will penetrate deeply into the tissues.

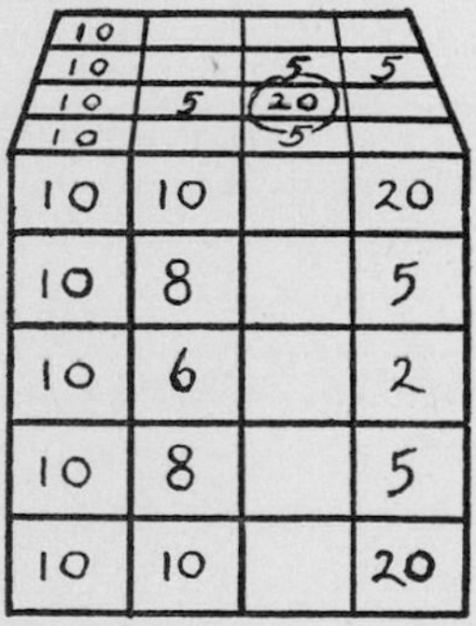

The cube represents possible distribution of short wave heating. Each square inch of surface area, and each cubic inch of deep tissue, should receive equal amounts of heat, instead of spotted and irregular heating. This is of course the ideal, seldom approached in actual treatment. Usually there is a thermal gradient from the hotter surface tissues to the less-heated deeper structures.

The problem of heat distribution in every case resolves itself into the following three considerations: (1) heat distribution on the skin surface, (2) penetrative heat, and (3) maintaining uniform distribution during treatment. In addition to electrical considerations it is necessary for the technician to give attention to special conditions that will affect the heat distribution, particularly anesthetized areas, and areas with poor circulation.

In order to help get more uniform distribution of surface heat with a maximum of penetrative heat, and with the penetration unchanging during the course of the treatment, the following simple rules may be observed for satisfactory application of condenser electrodes:

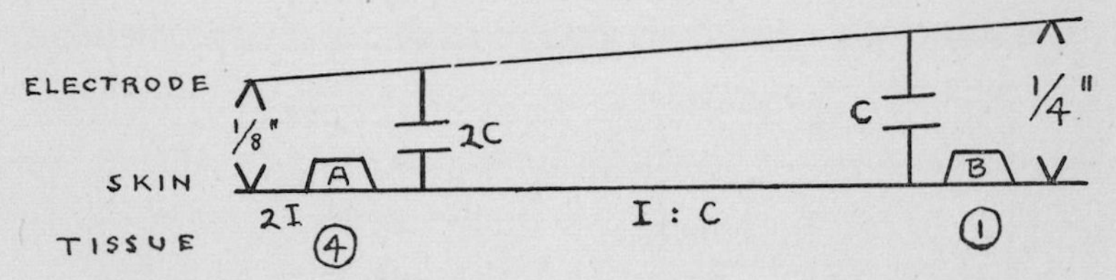

Diagram showing effects of irregular spacing of electrodes

1. Electrodes should be spaced uniformly from the skin. Irregular spacing produces spotted heating. For example, a square inch of skin surface A spaced ⅛ inch from the metal of an electrode will receive *twice* the amount of current as square inch B spaced ¼ inch from the electrode plate. Current (I) is inversely proportional to distance. But the two areas are heated in proportion to the *square* of the current. (Joule's Law: $W=I^2R$.) Therefore in the example cited the area A will receive *four times* as much heat as the area B. Increased total spacing will make for greater uniformity of surface heating.

2. Electrodes should be *adequately* spaced from skin. There is a need for substantial spacing of the electrode from the skin other than for its influence on uniformity of spacing. The factor of *penetration* is very largely controlled by E, the voltage of the induced electrical charge. A simplified diagram of the electrode circuit is shown,

C^1 and C^2 being the condenser electrodes. The portion of the body is represented by the capacity C^1 and the inductance g. The formula shown for heating is from DeWalt (*A Study of High Frequency Heating*). C is the capacity of the system; f is the frequency. The heating effect varies with the *square* of the voltage. The other values are *prime*. If the value of E is high enough to push the charge through

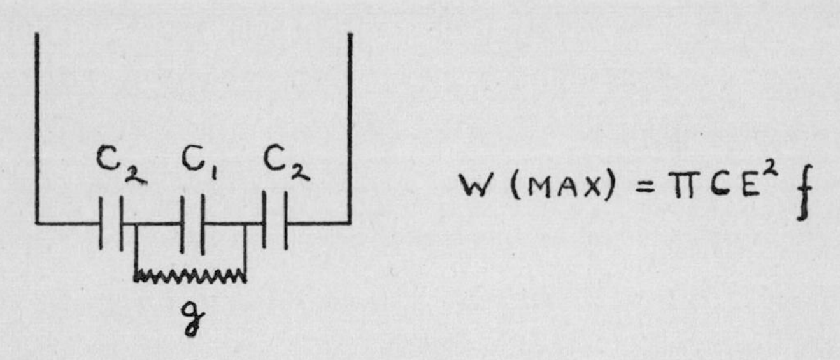

and through the patient, then maximum penetration results. If the value of E is lowered, surface heating increases. At a given wattage and wave-length, the closer the active part of the electrode is to the skin surface, the greater is the surface heating. Adequate spacing usually improves penetration.

3. The effect of accumulated perspiration should be watched carefully. Every treatment goes through three stages as far as perspiration is concerned.

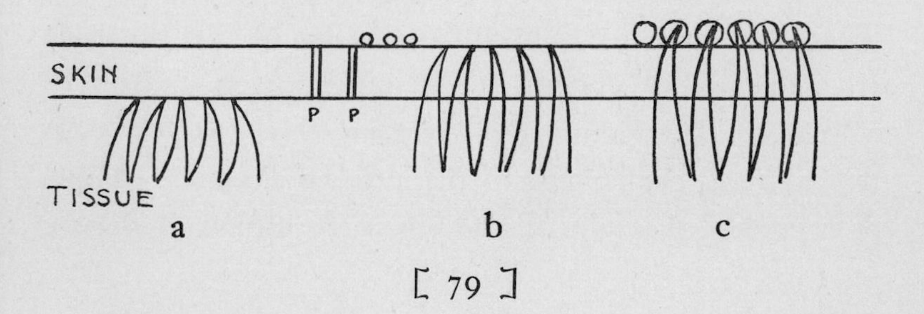

a. Skin is dry, with little or no heating in the skin. The dry skin offers too much resistance to the flow of the current.

b. Skin is moist, with lessened resistance, and increased heating.

c. Skin is saturated, perspiration has accumulated, and heating effects have now moved out into skin and perspiration. Unaided by the circulation possessed by deep tissues, the heating is cumulative, and, if long continued, might cause a burn.

The following suggestions will aid in the control of surface heating due to accumulating perspiration:

1. Turn the power almost all the way on at the start of the treatment, then *down* when comfortable warmth has been reached. A lower intensity will then maintain the warmth in the tissues, just as a low fire will maintain a constant temperature in a kettle of water after a high flame has been used to heat it.

2. Change towels if they become moistened.

3. Use shorter treatment times.

4. After initial heating, keep intensity of treatment *low*.

From time to time the question has arisen as to the relative merits of short wave apparatus as compared to "conventional" long wave apparatus. Clinically there may be no prominent difference in the results obtained from the two types of apparatus, but the question of preference has been very emphatically demonstrated by the almost complete disappearance from the market of the older type of machine. The convenience of short wave applications, the possible greater heating with deeper penetration, and the facility with which applications are made have appealed to the users.

PHYSICAL EFFECTS OF SHORT WAVE. Many controversial ideas have been expressed from time to time relative to the way in which the tissues are affected by the heating power of short waves. Several incorrect theories have been ad-

Fallacies about short wave heating

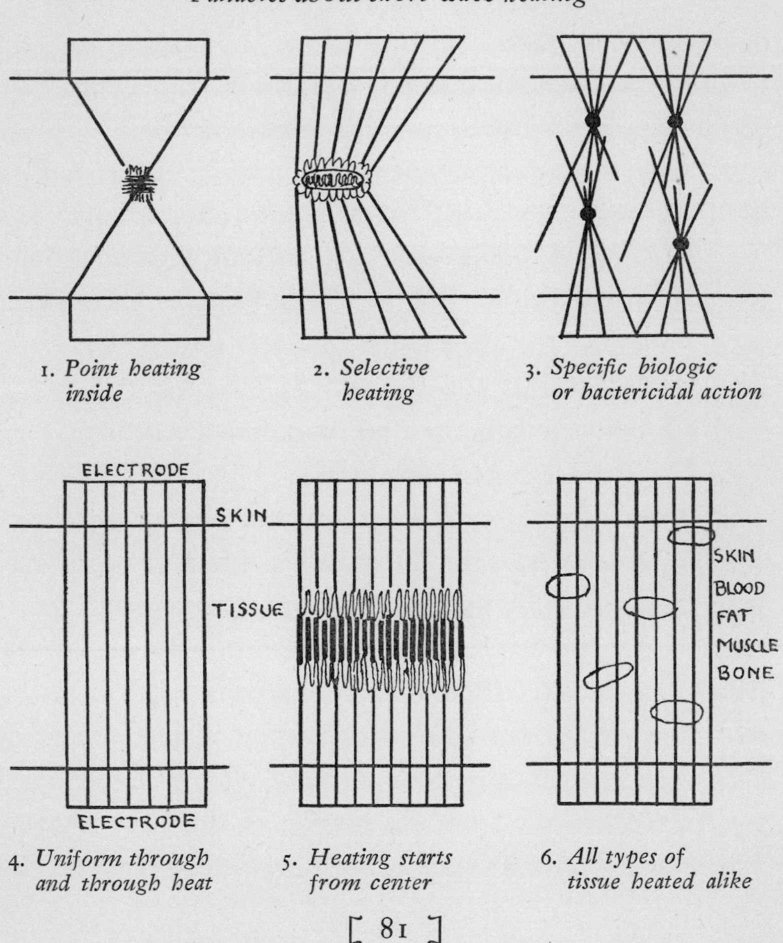

1. *Point heating inside*
2. *Selective heating*
3. *Specific biologic or bactericidal action*
4. *Uniform through and through heat*
5. *Heating starts from center*
6. *All types of tissue heated alike*

vanced, and much credence has been placed in one or more of these incorrect theories by reputable therapists. The preceding diagrams illustrate some of the fallacious ideas.

A careful study of the method by which the electrical losses are converted into heat shows that the heating does not follow a straight line path from electrode to electrode; that heating does not start in the center, and work outwardly; and that in the field between the electrodes the various types of body structure are not heated uniformly. Another fallacious idea carried over from an incorrect idea of the heating method of conventional diathermy is that of point heating, as illustrated in diagram No. 4. Nor has the idea of a selective heating of tissues been substantiated. As far as competent investigators have been able to ascertain, there is no demonstrable selective thermal action in the living body.

Certain specific effects on bacteria and their toxins have been claimed. No doubt these observations were confused with the results normally attributable to increased circulation and the hyperpyrexia produced. Short and ultra short wave radiation is biologically active only through the heat produced, and there is no authoritative evidence, so far, to show that there is any significance to high frequency treatments except that of heat. Claims of physiological effects in a large number of cases have not been substantiated.

There is no reason to believe that treatments of short duration, that is, five minutes or less, have any marked

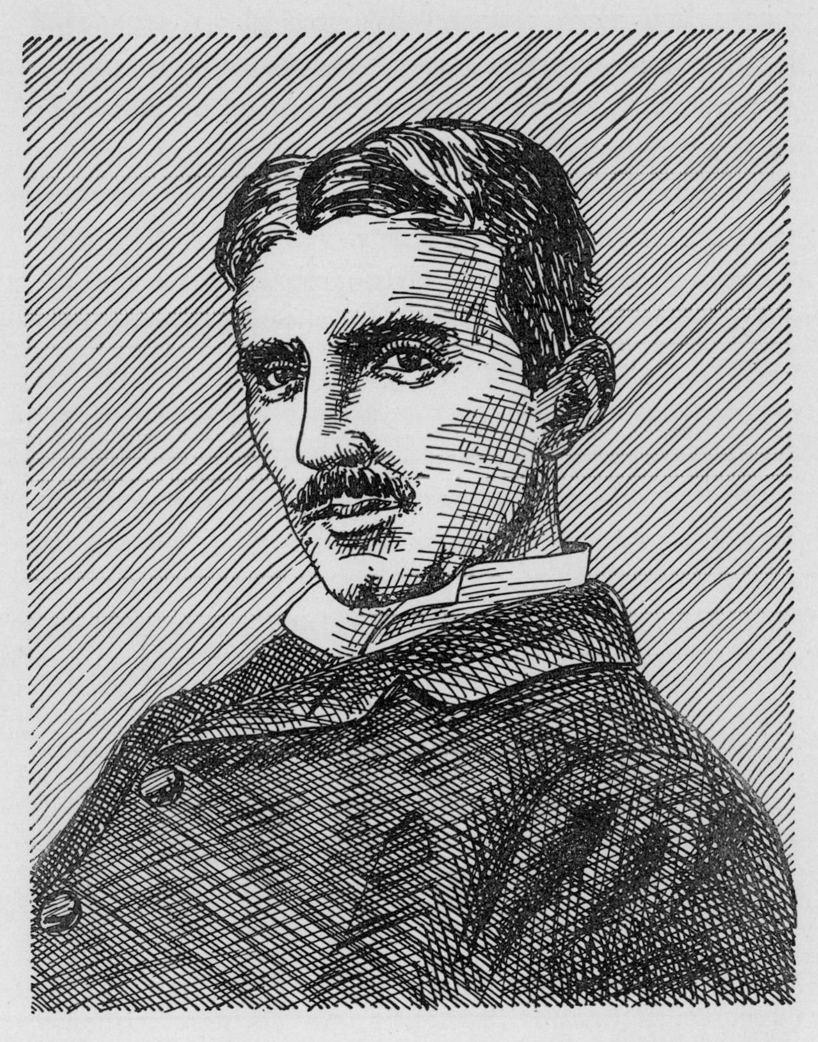

Nikola Tesla (1856-1943) was the first to suggest the possible therapeutic value of high frequency currents

action other than a psychic one; nor is there any authoritative evidence to substantiate the results claimed for therapeutic effects of very low intensity treatments, of intensity less than five watts. In reality the dosage should be applied according to the peculiar case of each patient, depending on the organ and nature of the disease. The sensitivity of various subjects is widely different. Some react to a very mild dosage, others to very strong ones. The present tendency seems to favor treatments from apparatus designed for high wattage output, with treatment intensities adjusted according to the tolerance or reaction of the patient. Efforts are being made toward greater facility of dosage contral, but the patient's own sensation is still the best and most effective guide.

BURNS. It is possible for burns to occur with short wave the same as with any type of thermal therapy. They can be completely avoided by the exercise of care in observing the few rules of application. The mere fact that electrodes are electrically insulated is not a guarantee against burns. Cords and electrodes should be well spaced from the body and from each other. If cords are allowed to touch, they may burn, melt, or char. Bed springs of the "inner-spring" type might easily become a menace and might be set afire by arcing of currents induced in the coils. Similarly, any metal between the electrode and the patient will pick up energy and may burn the patient. The hands of the patient or of the operator should not touch the electrodes during treatment, and the fingers should not touch the skin near the area being treated. The hand acts as any other conductor, and picks up energy from the field, which is harmless unless transferred to the body at a *point*, which will cause a burn.

Heating effects are cumulative during the treatment, and it is possible to burn a patient by over-treating, or by misjudging his tolerance to heat. Therefore, *never* leave the patient. *This is the best insurance against burns.* Safety must be the foremost consideration. There is no substitute for skill and *safety*.

The indications for use of short wave therapy should be considered to be the same as for the use of other types of heat therapy, which, in the majority of conditions, serves chiefly as an adjunct to other forms of treatment.

GENERAL SHORT WAVE OPERATING INSTRUCTIONS. Technical operation of the instrument will vary according to the type of machine in use, and therefore only basic electrode technic will be mentioned here.

The following methods of treatment application other than condenser electrodes are in general use:

1. Cuff electrodes. These are elongated condenser electrodes, designed to wrap around the extremities.

2. Induction cable. This method may be used with practically all machines, and in treating some parts of the body it is more easily applied than condenser plates. The same general rules apply for its safe use, as there is a capacity effect from the cable that might cause a burn.

3. Orificial electrodes, nonmetallic, and metallic. These electrodes produce the most efficient internal heating.

4. Drum electrodes, either inductive or capacitative.

There is no single method that is superior in all cases. Each method has certain inherent advantages, and each is capable of producing good results.

Always prepare the electrodes for each patient by wrapping each electrode in a clean cotton towel, and see that the cords are spaced well away from the body, and are well separated from each other.

The patient should be placed on a wooden treatment table or a well-insulated chair, treatment table, or couch. Do not use metal tables, and be sure that no metal is adjacent to the electrodes. Any metal or other conductor becomes highly charged in the field and may cause a slight burn to the patient or operator. The skin over the areas to be treated should be examined *before* and *after* treatment, and, except in rare cases, treatment should not be made through clothing. Watch carefully for articles of clothing that might contain metal threads, hidden pins, or clasps.

In general, place electrodes at nearly opposite sides of the parts to be treated. This is not a hard-and-fast rule, however, as often two electrodes are placed almost side by side, for example, in treatment of the spine.

When the patient is lying on one electrode it may be necessary to place more spacing between the electrode and the patient to equalize the heating. The basic rule to follow is: Place additional insulation (towels, rubber, etc.) under the warmer electrode, to equalize heating of the two electrodes.

A fundamental rule of diathermy is: "Select an active

electrode slightly smaller than the area to be treated." This suggests occasional use of small electrodes. It is obviously difficult to treat localized pathology, such as gall bladder, with large electrodes. One small electrode and one large electrode may be successfully employed with most short wave instruments.

SKIN RESISTANCE. High skin resistance, a limiting factor in metal-electrode diathermy, is of value in short wave diathermy because it tends to lessen surface heating. Accumulated perspiration lessens skin resistance, increases heat absorption, and should be avoided. Therefore it is sometimes advisable to start the treatment by turning the power *high* in order to get the maximum heating before perspiration has accumulated. Then turn the power almost all the way down, and build up again to tolerance.

INDIVIDUAL TOLERANCE. The guide for treatment intensity is individual tolerance. Careful observation of the time necessary to heat the various parts of the body, and of the intensity of the currents as indicated by the meter, will soon enable the operator to give treatments of desired intensity, with absolute safety.

DURATION OF TREATMENT. The time of each treatment with short wave apparatus will vary from ten minutes for each sinus application to twenty minutes for an average local treatment, up to thirty minutes and longer for chronic cases and treatment of deep-seated organs. When in doubt of patient's tolerance, start with ten-minute treatment, gradually increasing the time. Several hours' treatment is employed in hyperpyrexia.

HEAD AND NECK. Place one electrode between shoulders, held in place by patient resting against the electrode. Use a smaller active electrode adjacent to the part to be treated. This method may be used in treating sinus, antrum, ear, neck, or jaw. The cable is efficient for neck treatments.

SHOULDER. Place one large electrode between shoulders, a smaller electrode over the area to be heated, in such a position that the smaller electrode may be moved during treatment to alter the heating effects. The cable is best for shoulder applications.

FOOT. Place two large electrodes parallel, about three inches apart, on wooden floor or stool. Place foot on electrode, heel on one, toe on the other. Both feet may be treated at the same time.

LOWER LEG. Place one electrode on wooden floor, or other nonconductive surface, with at least a half inch or more of additional spacing between electrode and foot. Place the other electrode above patient's knee, with single towel spacing. The use of more spacing next to the foot lessens the heating in the ankle, makes it more pronounced higher up toward the knee.

KNEE. Extend the leg on treatment table and place one electrode under calf of leg, the other electrode immediately above the knee. Heating will be fairly uniform through the entire knee, with little heat noticeable adjacent to the electrodes. Cuff electrodes or cable are especially efficient.

WRIST, HANDS, FINGERS, LOWER ARM. Place two large electrodes on treatment table, about a foot apart, and have patient sit so that elbow may rest freely on one electrode.

Place the hand of the same arm on the other electrode. Heating will be apparent immediately in the wrist. To increase the heating in the hand and fingers, the palm of the fingers should be raised as far from the electrode as possible with the fingers still touching the electrode. This method will usually produce better heating than placing the hand between two electrodes.

In treating the hands and fingers it is sometimes helpful to remove the arm from the treatment field for a few minutes while the fingers are massaged; then return the arm to the field for further treatment.

BACK. Two pad electrodes on spine, about six inches apart. It is not necessary to have the electrodes on opposite sides of the body, as is often recommended.

ELBOW. With patient in sitting position, place one electrode adjacent to shoulder, with lower arm resting on other electrode.

HIP AND THIGH. Electrodes may be applied antero-posteriorly with the patient lying down.

CHEST. Treatment may be applied by condenser pads placed antero-posteriorly; or by a "pancake" coil placed over the chest. Do not permit patient to hold electrode or cable in place with hand unless pillow or other thick insulation is placed between hand and electrode.

ABDOMEN. Follow technic similar to chest. The electrode under the patient should be padded up more than the upper electrode, as the weight of the patient compresses the padding on the lower electrode, which increases heating.

MICROTHERMY

Recent utilization of the extremely short radio wave emanations of war-developed radar has provided a new therapeutic tool called microthermy. Wave lengths of microwaves are only 1/50th those of the six-meter ultra short waves. They are similar to the even shorter infra-red rays in that they may be reflected, and directed into a beam, or focused. Unlike infra red, however, they penetrate deeply into the tissues.

Claims to the effect that microthermy is a revolutionary new type of treatment have not been substantiated so far. No evidence has been produced to show that therapeutic effects have been due to anything other than heat, similar to the heating effects produced by conventional short wave apparatus.

Essentially, microthermy is "spotlight" application of diathermy energy, the application resembling both infra red, and the use of the drum applicator of short wave diathermy. Its particular usefulness is in the heat treatment of localized and irregular areas, such as sinuses, neck, ears, shoulders, knees, and hands. Since it is heat therapy, care must be exercised to prevent burns.

ELECTROSURGERY

The application of high frequency energy in sufficient intensity and concentration to produce destruction of tissue cells by cutting, coagulation, or desiccation is called *surgical diathermy*.

Coagulation electrodes may be monoterminal or biterminal. Cutting and desiccation electrodes are generally monoterminal.

The two factors which control the character of tissue destruction (i.e., whether by *cutting*, or heat-in-tissue destruction) are:

1. Concentration of energy. When continuous wave (undamped) high frequency energy is applied to tissue in sufficient intensity by means of knife-edge, point, or thin wire electrodes, the current advancing immediately ahead of the electrode cuts the tissue as quickly and as cleanly as does a sharp scalpel. If the area of the electrode is widened (for example, by applying the side of a knife-blade instead of the edge), coagulation of the tissues in contact with the blade results, without cutting.

2. Type of high frequency energy used. *Damped* currents of high frequency (of the type supplied by spark-gap apparatus) produce only coagulation or desiccation when concentrated at a knife-edge or pointed electrode.

Either damped or undamped currents may be employed in electrocoagulation if care is used in selecting the correct electrodes, but if both effects are desired from identical electrodes the two distinct types of currents should be available, either singly or "blended."

In electrocoagulation the destructive heat is produced within the tissues; in electrodesiccation the tissue is dehydrated by means of heat generated by sparks from the electrode.

REPRESENTATIVE WAVE LENGTHS

NATURE OF WAVE	CYCLES PER SECOND	WAVE LENGTH
Cosmic rays Received from interstellar space. Discovered by Millikan. Origin suspected to be associated with changes in atomic structure.	10^{21} - 10^{25}	.003 - .00003 AU
Gamma rays Emitted from radioactive substances.	10^{20}	.02 - .01 AU
X-rays Discovered by Roentgen. Produced by bombardment of matter by cathode particles in high vacuum.	10^{17} - 10^{18}	.01 - 5. AU
Ultra violet rays Produced by high pressure and low pressure electric arcs and by high temperature incandescent bodies.	10^{15} - 10^{16}	200 to 3900 AU
Visible light	4×10^{14} - 8×10^{14}	3900 AU - 7700 AU
Infra red (or heat rays) Produced by heated matter.	10^{11} - 4×10^{14}	7700 AU - .04 cm.
Microthermy (radar energy) Produced by cavity magnetron oscillators.	24×10^{8}	12 cm.
Ultra short wave diathermy Produced by tube oscillators.	5×10^{7}	6 meters
Short wave diathermy	2×10^{7}	15 meters
Conventional diathermy Produced by spark gap oscillators.	10^{6}	300 meters
House current Produced by mechanically powered electric generators.	60	5×10^{6} meters

Note: 1 AU (Angstrom Unit) equals 1/100,000,000th cm.

The electromagnetic spectrum as used in therapy

V

ELECTRODIAGNOSIS

EVER SINCE THE YEAR 1745 when Kratzenstein published the first report of muscle contraction resulting from stimulation with sparks from a frictional electricity generator, continued attempts have been made to study nerves and muscles of the body either by sending curents into these tissues, or by measuring the currents which the tissues produce in action. As progress has been made in methods of controlling the production of currents and in measuring and recording potential changes, dependable methods have been developed in the use of electrical phenomena in the study of nerves and muscles.

Electrodiagnosis may be defined as the utilization of electrical currents in the diagnosis of pathologic conditions of the body. The subject may be divided into two parts, depending on the origin of the electrical potentials:

1. The recording of results noted when muscles and nerves are stimulated by well-controlled externally applied electrical currents, and

2. The recording of electrical changes present in neuromuscular tissues, as is done in electrocardiography, electroencephalography, and electromyography.

It is the purpose of this discussion to describe some of the technics used only in the part of the subject of electrodiagnosis that concerns itself with externally applied electrical stimuli.

Early workers in the field of electrodiagnosis called attention to the fact that all parts and organs of the body are sensitive to electricity, and that this sensitivity may be modified by disease. Numerous handicaps, such as inadequate understanding of fundamental electrical currents, and lack of adequate experimental facilities to produce well-controlled stimuli, prevented accurate quantitative observations. Even with the recent development of electronic methods of investigation, the electrical phenomena of the nervous system are of such complexity that much progress is yet to be made before the part that changing electrical potentials play in affecting or indicating pathology is fully understood. Nerve currents may be exceedingly feeble; not only that, they may also be exceedingly brief. To record them has taxed the ingenuity of physiologists for years.

THE ELECTRICAL NATURE OF NERVES. Nerves transmit quantitative electrical information to the central nervous system about the parts and conditions of the body, and in the opposite direction they distribute signals initiating the finely graded activity of many organs. Many complex events occur as a result of this nerve activity, and the correct inauguration of all depends on the parts affected receiving the correct electrical signals by means of nerve transmission. Signals arranged in ever-changing patterns effectively convey all the information needed to produce coordinated activity of the many component parts of the body.

NERVE CONDUCTION. The whole process of nervous activity is not the simple transmission of an electrical current (like house current carried on a copper wire) from the brain to the part to be activated. Simple motor nerve conduction involves many processes. Unlike a single wire conductor, a motor nerve consists of a great many individual fibres, and may be described as being made up like a bundle of elongated, tubular, self-charging, "leaky" electrolytic condensers of varying diameter, all of which endeavor to go into action at the slightest provocation to contribute to coordinated and synchronized activity.

RECIPROCAL RELATIONSHIP BETWEEN NERVE AND MUSCLE. Any attempt to identify pathological changes in neuromuscular activity must take into consideration the reciprocal relationship existing between nerve and muscle tissue: (1) injury to or changes in nerve structure can alter the electrical signals, and thus change the metabolism and activation of the tissues supplied by the nerve, and (2) traumatic changes in the tissues may affect the nerve. It is here that the methods of electrodiagnosis step into the picture by attempting to measure the changes that take place in tissue as the result of pathology and interpreting these changes in terms of effects on the bodily mechanism as a whole.

COMPLEX NATURE OF NERVE ACTIVITY. There is evidence to show that the following occurrences are associated with activity in nervous tissue:

1. An increase in metabolism.
2. An increase in heat production.
3. An alteration of excitability.
4. An alteration of electrical impedence.

5. A sequence of electrical potential changes.

With pathology there is a general slowing down of all these activities.

DUPLICATION OF ACTION IMPULSES. An approach to the subject of electrodiagnosis from the standpoint of externally applied stimuli has a logical start if an attempt is made to identify the nature of normal action potentials, isolate the individual "action unit," and then substitute an artificial action unit similar to the normal one, but with variable and controllable characteristics to be used to stimulate the areas suspected of having pathology or pathological tendencies.

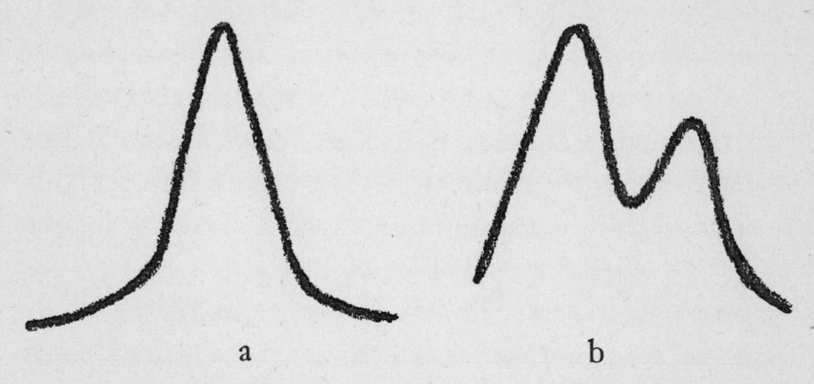

Oscillogram of (a) *motor unit* (b) *sensory unit*

VARIETY OF METHODS USED. Several methods of electrodiagnosis have been employed, all of which record changes that take place in factors that determine the shape and position of the strength-duration curve, such as changes in intensity, changes in duration, and changes in rate of acceleration of the threshold stimulus. Examples of these methods are the galvanic method, the faradic method, the condenser test, the method of chronaxy, the skin-resistance test, the sinusoidal method, and a high frequency method that has been used in England. There is also the tetanus-twitch ratio test which attempts to measure changes in accommodation. Actually there is little basic difference in these various methods; the differences that do exist arise because no one method utilizes all the facts necessary to make a complete diagnostic picture. There must be a correlation of all the methods. The key to the situation lies with the individual *action impulse*, with accurate determinations of the factors of time and amplitude. In the light of recent investigations, the effects of stimuli of various durations and amplitudes can be anticipated accurately.

THE MOTOR POINT. Before getting into the technic of muscle testing it might be well to mention the keynote of electrodiagnosis—the motor point. This is the projection on the surface of the skin at the point where the nerve divides into the underlying muscle tissue, and at a distance from the penetration of the nerve into the muscle, varying with the muscle. Bourguignon's demonstration of the true motor point of the muscle shows that in normal muscles the threshold response is evoked only by excitation of the nerves.

CLASSICAL METHODS. In actual practice the long-established methods of galvanic-faradic testing are not sufficiently accurate to meet present-day demands because they identify only the two extremes of irritability. The familiar polar formula KCC>ACC>AOC>KOC indicates only whether extreme degeneration exists, but not to what degree. The test is chiefly qualitative.

SYNOPSIS OF REACTIONS OF DEGENERATION (R.D.)

ABSOLUTE	*Nerve and muscle*	No response to any form of electrical excitation
COMPLETE	*On the nerve*	Loss of excitation, galvanic and faradic
	On the muscle	Loss of faradic excitation *Slow* response to galvanic or diminished response Galvanotonus Equalization or inversion of formula Longitudinal reaction
PARTIAL	*On the nerve*	Diminished excitation to faradism and galvanism
	On the muscle	Faradic response diminished Galvanic response first increased[1] then diminished, also *slow* Galvanotonic reaction Longitudinal reaction
TRACE	*On nerve and muscle*	Faradic and galvanic excitation almost normal Galvanism produces normal excitation on K.C.C., slow on A.C.C.

[1]This is often missed.

STRENGTH-DURATION CURVES. For better study of excitability of nerves and muscles the factors of current strength, duration, and increase of potential must be considered. Electric impulse generators are now available that have these factors accurately under control. With instantaneously applied impulses of the condenser-discharge or square-wave types, it has been found that a definite relationship exists between the duration and strength of the impulse necessary to elicit a threshold response. By varying these factors it is possible to plot a curve, called the strength-duration curve, which gives a graphic picture of the state of nerve and muscle excitability. Changes in the position and shape of the curve denote corresponding changes in nerve fibres and muscle structure.

TYPE OF CONTRACTION. In dealing with the question of muscle response to electrical stimuli certain characteristics are of clinical importance: (1) the nature of the contraction—is it brisk or slow? and (2) the amplitude of the contraction—is it normal or diminished? In the case of sensory nerves, the qualitative reaction is the nature of the sensation evoked, and the direction of its propagation. These factors can be ascertained with any good apparatus supplying galvanic and faradic currents, but such instrumentation is limited strictly to qualitative results.

ACCURACY IN DETERMINATIONS. The absolute *measurement* of excitability resulted from the discovery of Hoorveg and Weiss of the laws of excitation. The method of measurement was improved by Lapicque, who first established the principles of chronaxy in animals. Bourguignon improved the application of the principles to human beings.

CHRONAXIMETRY. Chronaxy (or chronaxie) is a term introduced by Louis Lapicque in 1909 to define the character of a stimulus which is required to excite various types of living tissue, particularly muscle and nerve. (*Excite* is used in the sense that a tissue is caused to display its characteristic activity.) The most convenient form of a stimulus, as we have seen, is an electrical impulse, since this can be made to excite the tissue without doing any damage, and can be accurately measured and reproduced. Other types of stimuli might be used, such as percussion, pressure, chemical application, and heat, but would harm the tissues.

REQUIREMENTS OF STIMULUS. In order to excite tissue an electrical impulse must fulfill the following conditions:

1. It must reach a certain amplitude.
2. It must have at least a minimum duration.
3. The *rate of increase* from zero to maximum must exceed a certain value. A gradually increased impulse will not evoke a muscular contraction.

The need for a minimum duration is shown by the fact

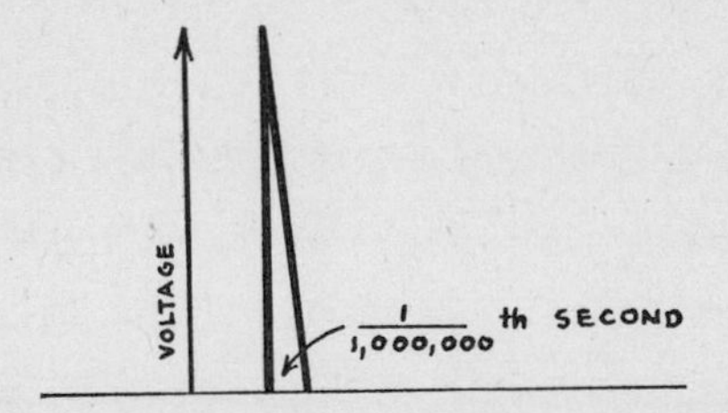

Electrical impulse of extremely short duration elicits no contractile stimulation

that rapidly oscillating currents (above 1,000,000 cycles per second) are powerless to excite any tissue of the human body. Modern diathermy makes use of this fact in the application of relatively large currents of high frequency energy for the purpose of producing heat within the tissue, without causing sensory or contractile effects.

STRENGTH-DURATION CURVE. The curve showing the relationship between minimum duration and minimum intensity is shown in the illustration. It is known as the strength-duration curve. Lapicque established the fact that the time measurement (chronaxy) expressed all the functional properties of the nerve and muscle, hence its extreme importance. Lapicque has also shown that curves of the same form are obtainable from the most diverse tissue, ranging from the human nerve, where the duration is as short as .0001 second, to the cells of a plant, where it may be longer than 1 second.

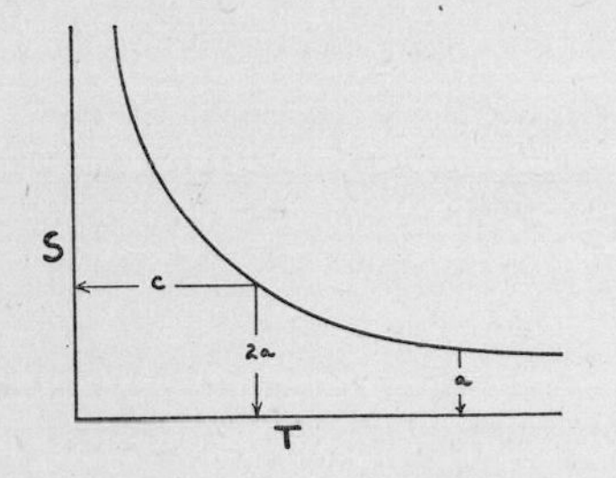

The curve shows the relation between the strength and duration of the smallest current that will excite a living cell. The chronaxy (c) *and the rheobase* (a) *are the two constants which define the curve.*

Form of stimulating current in living tissue

As a first approximation the curve obeys the formula of Weiss, I=a plus b/t, where I is current, t is time, and a and b are constants. Thus the character of a stimulus for a given tissue can be defined at once if we know the constants for the tissue. The constant a is the rheobase, which may be defined as the minimum intensity of "square wave" impulse of long duration that will cause a threshold contraction. The other constant is more important, for it determines the slope of the curve. It can be determined by measuring the chronaxy, which is equal to b/a, and is the least duration required when the current is of 2a intensity.

The true form of the curve differs somewhat from that given by Weiss' equation, and it has been used as a basis from which to deduce the mechanism of excitation. In Lapicque's hands chronaxy has also been used to investigate the passage of the state of excitation from one tissue to another (i.e., from nerve to muscle).

By the use of repeated determinations of such strength-duration curves the progressive changes in irritability of both motor and sensory nerves, and of muscles, can be measured; the evolutions of lesions of a degenerative character may be followed with a degree of precision.

Chronaxy plays an important role in both diagnosis and prognosis, and it indicates and regulates the therapy. Prior to the discovery of chronaxy it was difficult to accomplish this. Even in a temporary injury of a muscle the chronaxy may change from one-third to ten times normal, although from the galvanic-faradic tests the type of contraction would still be brisk and would be passed as normal.

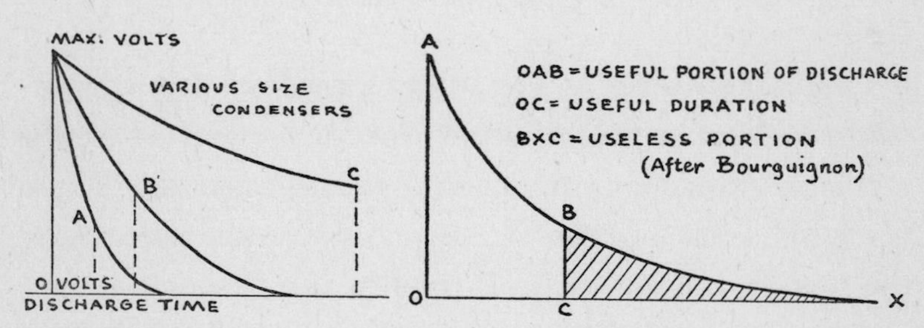

Diagrams illustrating the use of various size condenser discharges to obtain accurately timed impulses

BOURGUIGNON'S LAWS OF CHRONAXY

1. The chronaxy of a healthy muscle is the same as that of the nerve, on the motor point, and by longitudinal excitation. (A pathological muscle is heterogeneous.)

2. In a segment of a limb the chronaxy is the same for all muscles of the same function.

3. For the same function the muscles of the proximal

segment have a smaller chronaxy than those in the distal segment in the ratio of 1:2.5.

In considering the muscles as a whole the distribution of their chronaxies is a functional distribution, not correlated with anatomical positions.

From a medical viewpoint Bourguignon has shown that all the nerves and muscles in the same region that have the same chronaxies not only have the same function, but are predisposed to the same pathology. Bourguignon used chronaxy as a means for the study of the whole nervous system, which he viewed as a vast system of resonance in which the normal and pathological excitations reverberate according to resonances revealed by the measurement of chronaxy values.

CHRONAXY VALUES. The values for various normal muscles have been very carefully worked out, and they are remarkably constant from one individual to another. There is a fairly constant ratio of 2 to 1 between the muscles on the posterior aspect of an extremity and those on its anterior aspect, while the proximal segments of a limb have a shorter chronaxy than the distal segments.

SIGNIFICANCE OF UNIT VALUES. For the proximal regions, the anterior muscles show a range of from .06 to .14 sigma, the posterior from .16 to .34 sigma; for the distal regions the values for the anterior muscles are from .40 to .70. Thus, for all practical purposes, all values over 1 unit chronaxy (1 sigma) can be considered pathological. In cases which show the complete "reaction of degeneration" the chronaxy is generally found to be from 10 to 20 sigma,

FORM OF CONTRACTION	CHRONAXY	PATHOLOGIES		
Brisk contraction	⅓ to 5 x normal	Repercussions	Lesion of a nerve (mixed)	Permanent modifications
			Lesion of sensitive peripheric neurone	
			Lesion of central neurones	
			Atrophies (reflex)	
		Irritation		
		Beginning of degeneration		
		Lowering of temperature		Temporary modifications
		Vaso-motor troubles		
Slow to de-contract	5 to 15 x normal	Wallerian degeneration		Permanent modifications
Galvanotonus beginning brisk	10 x normal to 9 sigma	Myopathy		
Galvanotonus beginning slow	9 to 20 sigma	Thomsen's disease		
Contraction very slow	20 to 40 sigma	Lowering of temperature		Temporary modifications
Contraction myotonic	40 to 80 sigma	Vaso-motor troubles		

From *Electricity in Therapeutics* by H. H. U. Cross, London, 1936 while in cases of muscular dystrophy values as high as 80 may be encountered. Thus we see that the definitely abnormal values are so far removed from their normal range as to make their recognition certain, and changes may be recognized long before they would become apparent with the methods commonly used to determine the reaction of degeneration.

CHRONAXY OF INFANTS. Infants at birth have greater chronaxy values for both nerves and muscles than adults. At about the second or third month the chronaxy of the nerves is normal, but that of the muscles is excessively high. At walking age the child's chronaxy values are about the same as an adult's, with the chronaxy of nerves and their muscles the same.

TOTAL SECTION OF NERVE. When the nerve is totally sectioned the whole nerve degenerates, and all the muscles have approximately the same large chronaxy values. The muscle is said to be in a state of total degeneration.

PARTIAL SECTION OF NERVE. The same does not apply when the nerve is only partially sectioned, or only partially affected by a pathological process. In this case, two chronaxies can be found, one normal or nearly so, which is found at the motor point, and which remains partially excitable; the other, of greater value than normal, by longitudinal excitation. Here is found the so-called partial degeneration, in which only certain fibres of a muscle are affected and because of which a portion of the muscle is degenerated, the remainder being in a healthy, normal condition.

SEQUENCE OF DEGENERATIVE CHANGES. When it is possible to follow the degenerative process from its inception, there is first a short phase in which the chronaxy may descend to ½ or ⅓ of the normal, then a progressive increase without much visible evidence by way of alteration in character of the contraction. By the time the chronaxy becomes ten times normal, the contraction begins to slow until anywhere between 10 and 70 it is seen at its slowest. If at this stage regeneration does not take place, then the chronaxy redescends a little where it remains until the disappearance of all excitability.

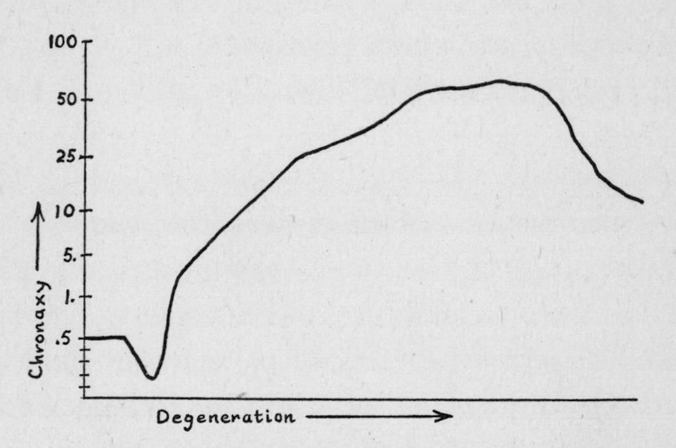

Diagram illustrating changing chronaxy values with degenerative changes

In chronaxy testing, care must be exercised in locating the motor point, as well as in the observation of the threshold contractions, which are used as the basic unit of intensity (rheobase). However, evaluation of the speed and type of contraction, so important in other methods, is not essential, being merely confirmatory of objective findings.

NATURE OF OBJECTIVE DETERMINATIONS. In chronaxy testing it is necessary to record only the numerical chronaxy values, which reflect a measure of the state of total irritability of tissue. However, an instrument designed for chronaxy testing can be used to make the following determinations:

1. Location of motor point.
2. Degree of faradic excitability.
3. Rheobase (galvanic excitability).
4. Galvanic sensory irritability.
5. Polarity reactions, whether the reactions to the polar formula are normal, equal, or reversed.
6. Type of contraction (brisk, slow, slow to decontract, etc.).
7. Chronaxy.
8. Other points on strength-duration curve.

WARM MUSCLES AND MOIST SKIN NECESSARY. Hydration of the skin increases electroconductivity. Warming of muscles increases their irritability and contractility. Before electrically testing, or before stimulating weak and degenerated muscles, they should be warmed.

TECHNIC OF CHRONAXY TESTING. The first step in chronaxy testing is to seek out those muscles that are pathologic. A short-cut may be used by taking advantage of the old rule: "try the faradic first." This may be done by setting the chronaxy impulse of the instrument at .25, with the voltage dial setting as maximum. The result is a sharply peaked "faradic unit" that will momentarily contract almost all normal muscles, without the tetany and pain that would result from the application of a faradic current of the same intensity. Muscles that contract briskly may be eliminated at once from consideration. Where a muscle fails to respond it is marked for further study. A chart should be compiled, with the names of the suspected nerves and muscles, and with spacing for the recording of several tests to be made at regular intervals. Preliminary elimination of normal muscles from the complete test saves a great deal of time and lessens the danger of fatigue to both patient and operator.

MUSCLE-NERVE TEST CHARTS. Prepared charts similar to those illustrated for all parts of the body save a great deal of time in recording results of chronaxy tests. They show the approximate motor and nerve areas, the name of each motor nerve and each muscle, the function of each muscle, and the chronaxy value of the normal, according to Bourguignon. The charts may also be used to indicate the placement of electrodes for therapy. Of course it is not necessary to run a chronaxy test on every nerve and muscle just to fill all the spaces. Absence of a notation for any muscle means it was not found to have lessened irritability on the initial "faradic" test. The possible danger of relying exclusively on the faradic test is that it fails to show the earliest stage of denervation, without an element of time intervening.

Progressive changes in the chronaxy values will indicate whether improvement is being made as a result of therapeutic measures applied. In many cases the course of such changes will be shown long before they are confirmed by objective responses.

TYPE	TIME AFTER ONSET OF FACIAL PALSY				
	ONE WEEK	TWO WEEKS	THREE WEEKS	FOUR WEEKS	SIX WEEKS
CLINICAL	Complete paralysis	Complete paralysis	Forehead improved	Foreh'd good; mouth slightly improved	Almost normal
FRONTALIS	.28	12.	6.	1.2	.8
ORBICULARIS	.6	9.2	8.8	6.8	1.

This is an example of the correlation between clinical improvement and change in chronaxy values.

CHRONAXY ELECTRODES. The dispersive electrode can be any convenient size, preferably about 4″ x 6″. It is best always to use the same size, for standardization of results. The well-moistened pad of the electrode should be in firm contact with the back or chest. Place the electrode in midline when comparing both sides.

The active electrode should be light weight, about one half inch in diameter, covered with moisture-retaining material, and attached to a rigid electrode holder about 7 or 8 inches in length. The electrode must be well moistened at all times during the test. After the motor point is located, the electrode must be kept in the same position and at the same pressure throughout the rest of the test on that point. A variation in the size of the electrode will make very little difference in the chronaxy readings, but the small electrode helps to limit the stimulus to a single motor point. The negative pole is always connected to the active electrode at the start of the test.

METHOD OF TESTING. An increasing intensity of current is applied to the motor point, interruptedly, until the muscle contracts. This is called the rheobase, or threshold of contraction. The current is then applied at double-rheobase intensity for increasing periods until a contraction is elicited. The minimum duration of the double-rheobase intensity impulse that will cause a threshold contraction denotes the chronaxy of the muscle. It is recorded in sigma, a sigma being 1/1000th second of double-rheobase current. All normal values for skeletal muscles are less than 1 sigma.

THE USE OF CHRONAXY DETERMINATIONS

MOTOR NERVE DIAGNOSIS. The segment of a nerve distal to a peripheral nerve lesion will not conduct current. The chronaxy determinations in such instances are really of the muscles themselves. Most muscles with intact nerves will have a chronaxy of less than 1 sigma. The degree of degeneration can thus be diagnosed.

ANTERIOR HORN CELL DISEASE. If a sufficient number of anterior horn cells are diseased, the muscles supplied by them will have large chronaxy values.

SENSORY NERVE DIAGNOSIS. Impairment of sensory nerves will give increased chronaxy readings.

NERVE REPAIR PROGNOSIS. The appearance or reappearance of normal chronaxy presages return of function.

Chronaxy represents an easily obtainable index of the functional state of nerve and muscle which can be gained in no other manner, and provides a quantitative and objective measure of the functional state which is not possible in other methods of diagnosis. It is, of course, difficult to grasp at first the terms of rheobase, chronaxy, and strength-duration curves, but an understanding of such fundamental concepts is necessary because of their importance in the diagnosis and prognosis of neuromuscular conditions.

The chief advantage of the method of chronaxy is that it gives all the facts about muscle function, in spite of variations in intensity of stimulus from muscle to muscle, and in the same muscle from time to time. The principal disadvantage of chronaxy is that it fails to establish evidence of earliest reinnervation. When reinnervation begins to occur some fibres will receive their innervation before others. So there are really two curves. The tetanus-twitch ratio test recognizes the existence of these two curves in establishing evidence of reinnervation. It would be an ideal method if it did not take so much time, requiring as much as half an hour per muscle.

With the use of modern electronic testing instruments, and with simplified procedures, well-charted tests can be made rapidly and accurately by a competent physical therapy technician without the necessity of the doctor's taking his valuable time to run the test. The use of specially prepared muscle and nerve test charts greatly facilitates the preparation of reliable and pertinent chronaxy reports.

The muscle-nerve test charts shown on pages 126-129 have been reduced to book page size for illustrative purposes.

VI
LOW VOLTAGE TREATMENT CHART

THE FOLLOWING COMPILATION of galvanic and contractile current treatment data is offered as a quick and ready reference for treatment applications. The variety of treatments shown indicates the versatility of a modern low voltage treatment instrument.

Changes in the technics outlined may be made in conformity with the technician's own interpretations of the conditions encountered, and to suit individual requirements. The chart is suggested as a method of classification of treatment data rather than as a system of therapy. New technics may be outlined in *one line* of the chart with the aid of abbreviations, and the record will serve as a *starting point* for subsequent similar treatments. In some conditions several approaches to the problem are suggested.

In considering the problem of dosage, the values listed are *maximal*. The rules of tolerance must not be exceeded at any time. In galvanic treatments ½ ma. per square inch of the smaller electrode is a safe intensity to use for all applications, in no instances exceeding 1 ma. per square inch except in the treatment of mucous surfaces where the intensity of current used often may be greater. It is better to take a longer treatment time than to use excessive amounts of current.

With the contractile currents, contraction of the muscles, or sensation of pain (if produced) are the only reliable guides. Please note that there is no substitute for experience on the part of the operator with the apparatus being used, and it is safer to undertreat until one is thoroughly familiar with the equipment.

ABBREVIATIONS USED. Each of the twelve columns of the chart contain words and abbreviations as explained below:

1. Name of condition, disease, or part to be treated.

2. The immediate objective of the treatment, with abbreviations of the following:

Absorption	Massage
Coagulation	Mobilization
Decongestion	Nerve or muscle stimulation
Disinfection	Muscle exercise
Desensitization	Relaxation
Dilation	Relief of pain
Exercise	Softening
Electrical massage	Sterilization
Fungicidal action	Stimulation
Hemostasis	Tonic
Ionization	Vasodilation

3. Current selected. Applies to active electrode if the effect is to be localized.

Galvanic current numerals G-1, G-2, etc. indicate the particular use of the current, as follows:

G-1. To introduce drugs into superficial tissues.
G-2. To alleviate pain.
G-3. To stimulate the nervous system.

G-4. To soften scar and other tissue.
G-5. To increase bactericidal or fungicidal action.
G-6. To produce local destruction of tissue.
G-7. To control bleeding.
G-8. To dilate restricted passages.

Contractile currents, C-1, C-2, etc. Disregard numerals if using single-frequency instruments. Please note that the function of all contractile currents is the production of muscular contractions, and therapeutic results may be produced by a large number of currents, of many frequencies. The numerals denote the first choice of the following frequency ranges:

C-1. Higher frequencies, 100 to 2,500, of which the faradic is an example. They produce intense tetanic-type contractions.

C-2. Medium-frequency range currents, of approximately 40 to 100 per second. This rate matches approximately the normal innervation of vigorous skeletal muscle activity.

C-3. Lower frequency currents, with a range of approximately 10 to 40 per second, with extended "action units," for stimulation of partially denervated muscles, involuntary muscles, or deep-seated muscle groups.

C-4. "Static" discharge currents, consisting of spaced individual impulses, each impulse producing a distinct contraction. The frequency range is below 5 per second.

Sup. Superimposed, also called pulsating galvanic, combines galvanic and contractile effects. The frequency range may be anywhere from 60 per second to 2,500 per second.

4. & 5. Electrodes. Columns 4 and 5 indicate size and placement of the electrodes, listing that of the active electrode if current is to be concentrated there; otherwise both electrodes are considered active, but of opposite polarity in galvanic applications.

Electrode size. Because of many sizes in use the following designations have been made:

Point. A ball or disc, up to 2″ in diameter.

Small. From 2 sq. inches to 10 sq. inches in area (ex. 2″ x 3″).

Medium. 10 sq. in. to 20 sq. in. (example 3″ x 5″).

Large. More than 20 sq. in. in area. (example 4″ x 8″).

Placement. Areas of placement are indicated by abbreviation of such terms as pathology, lesion, muscle, motor points, dorsal, lumbar, abdomen, gall bladder, etc. When the same area is designated for both electrodes they should be placed side by side, about two inches apart.

6. & 7. The same as above for patient's outlet #2. This is usually the indifferent (or dispersive) electrode.

8. Intensity. The values are *maximum*, not to be exceeded.

   a. Galvanic intensity indicated in milliamperes.

   b. Contractile intensity indicated by degree of contractile activity, such as SC, sub-contractile; MC, mild contractions; and IC, intense contractions.

9. Surge timing. The numbers denote the approximate number of surges per minute. Zero (0) denotes continuous (nonsurging) current.

10. Recommended maximum treatment time *in minutes*.

11. Frequency. The number of treatments *per week* that may be given with safety. 3 means three treatments per week, on alternate days. D (daily) or 6 denotes treat every day.

12. Solutions, if any, that may be used. Some of the abbreviations are for the following: histamine, mecholyl, copper sulphate, copper, zinc, sodium chloride, etc. Adjunctive treatments, such as short wave, may be listed also.

COND.	AIM	CUR.	ELEC.	PLACE	ELEC.	PLACE	SURGE	INTEN.	TIME	FREQ.	SOLS.
Adhesions—Musc. (1)	Soften	G-4-N	Med.	Path.	Lge.	Ind.	0	15	15	1-2	NaCl
Adhesions—Musc. (2)	Exerc.	C-2	Med.	Path.	Lge.	Spine	20	MC	5-10	3-6	
Adhesions—Abd.	Mass.	C-3	Med.	7-8 D	Med.	7-8 D	12-15	IC	5-15	3-6	
Abscess	Disinf.	G-5-P	Med.	Lesion	Lge.	Ind.	0	10-20	10	2-3	ZnSO4
Adenitis (1)	Decong.	G-1-N	Med.	Path.	Lge.	Ind.	0	10-20	15-20	2-3	KI
Adenitis (2)	Decong.	C-3	Med.	Path.	Lge.	Ind.	20-30	MC	5-10	3-6	
Ankylosed joints (1)	Mobil.	G, N & P	Lge.	Joint	Lge.	Ind.	0	10-20	20-40	2	Mec.
Ankylosed joints (2)	Mobil.	C-3	Med.	Musc.	Lge.	Ind.	15-20	MC	10	3-6	
Arthritis, acute	Pn. Rel.	G-3	Lge.	Path.	Lge.	Ind.	0	10-20	10-20	2-3	
Arthritis, chronic (1)	Stim.	C-3-4	Lge.	Path.	Lge.	Ind.	20	MC	5-15	3-6	
Arthritis, chronic (2)	Decon.	G-1-P	Lge.	Joint	Lge.	Path.	0	10-20	10-20	2	Mec.
Athlete's foot	Fung.	G-5	Basin	Foot	Lge.	Ind.	0	10-15	10-15	2-3	CuSO4
Bruises	Decon.	Sup.-P	Med.	Path.	Lge.	Ind.	30	10-15	10	2	
Buerger's	Stim.	C-2-3	Lge.	Extrem.	Lge.	Extrem.	20-30	MC	10-20	3-6	

COND.	AIM	CUR.	ELEC.	PLACE	ELEC.	PLACE	SURGE	INTEN.	TIME	FREQ.	SOLS.
Bursitis	Decon.	C-2	Med.	Burs.	Lge.	Ind.	15-20	MC	10-15	3-6	
Colitis (1)	Stim.	Sup.-N	Lge.	Abd.	Lge.	Back	12	20	10-15	2-3	
Colitis (2)	Stim.	C-3	Lge.	Abd.	Lge.	Back	12	MC	10-15	3-6	
Cholycystitis	Decon.	C-3	Med.	G.B.	Lge.	Ind.	15	MC	5-10	3-6	
Cervix (1)	Coag.	G-6-P	Orif.	Cerv.	Lge.	Ind.	0	15-20	15-20	1	Cu
Cervix (2)	Dilate	G-8-N	Orif.	Cerv.	Lge.	Ind.	0	10	10	2-3	
Earache	Pn. Rel.	G-1-P	Orif.	Ear	Med.	Ind.	0	2-5	10-20	2-3	$ZnSO_3$
Fibroids	Reduce	G-4-N	Sm.	Path.	Lge.	Ind.	0	10-20	15-30	2	Cu
Fibrositis	Stim.	G-3	Med.	Path.	Lge.	Ind.	0	10-20	10-15	2	Mec.
Fistula	Ion.	G-6-P	Zn Wire	Fist.	Lge.	Ind.	0	10	10	1	Zn
Fractures	M. Stim.	C-2	Med.	Path.	Lge.	Path.	20-30	MC	5-10	2-3	
Foot	M. Stim.	C-2	Med.	Ball	Med.	Heel	20	IC	10	3-6	
Goitre	Ion.	G-1-N	Med.	Path.	Lge.	Ind.	0	10	15	2	KI
Gastroptosis	Stim.	C-3	Med.	Epig.	Lge.	Ind.	15	IC	10-15	3-6	

COND.	AIM	CUR.	ELEC.	PLACE	ELEC.	PLACE	SURGE	INTEN.	TIME	FREQ.	SOLS.
Hay Fever	Desen.	G-6	Pack	Nose	Lge.	Ind.	0	3-8	15	1	$ZnSO_4$
Hemorrhage, uterine	Hem. Sta.	G-7-P	Orif.	Uter.	Lge.	Ind.	0	10-25	15-30	1	Cu
Hem., Keesey (1)	Coag.	G-6-N	Needle	Pile	Lge.	Ind.	0	10-	10-	1-2	
Hem. (2)	Shrink	G-6-P	Orif.	Rect.	Lge.	Ind.	0	15	15	1	Cu
Hemiplegia	Stim.	C-3	Sm.	Musc.	Med.	Ind.	20	MC	5-10	3-6	
Hiccough (1)		C-4	Med.	Epigas.	Lge.	Back	0	IC	10-20	D	
Hiccough (2)	N. Exc.	C-1	Med.	Phrenic	Lge.	Ind.	45	MC	20-30	D	
Hypertension	N. Sed.	C-2	2 Lge.	Calves	Lge.	Liver	15	MC	15-20	3-6	
Intestinal Stasis	Stim.	C-3 G-N	Lge.	Abd.	Lge.	Back	20	IC	10-20	3-6	
Liver	Stim.	C-3	Med.	Epigas.	Lge.	5-7 Th	15	IC	10-15	2-3	
Lumbago	N. Sed.	G-1	Med.	Path.	Lge.	Ind.	0	10	15	2-3	
Migraine	Pn. Rel.	G-1-P	Med.	Pain	Lge.	Sol. Plex.	0	10-15	10-15	2-3	
Neuritis (1)	N. Sed.	G-1-P	Lge.	Path.	Lge.	Path.	0	15-25	20-30	3	
Neuritis (2)	N. Sed.	C-1	Lge.	Path.	Lge.	Ind.	30-40	SC	30	D	

COND.	AIM	CUR.	ELEC.	PLACE	ELEC.	PLACE	SURGE	INTEN.	TIME	FREQ.	SOLS.
Neuritis (3)	N. Sed.	C-2	Lge.	Path.	Lge.	Ind.	20-30	MC	20	3-6	
Obesity	Musc. Ex.	C-2	Lge.	Musc.	Lge.	Musc.	30-45	IC	20-40	3-6	
Optic atrophy	N. Stim.	G-3-N	Pack	Eyes	Med.	Neck	0	2-5	5-15	2-3	
Paralysis (1)	N. Stim.	G-3-N	Lge.	Path.	Lge.	Ind.	0	10-20	10-15	2-3	
Paralysis (2)	M. Stim.	C-3	Pt.	Musc.	Med.	Ind.	20-30	MC	10	3-6	
Prolapse (1)	Shrink	G-6-P	Orif.	Rect.	Lge.	Ind.	0	15	10-15	1-2	Cu
Prolapse (2)	Stim.	C-2	Orif.	Rect.	Lge.	Ind.	30	MC	10-15	3-6	
Prostate (1)	Decon.	C-4	Orif.	Rect.	Lge.	Ind.	15	IC	10-15	3-6	
Prostate (2)	Decon.	G-5-P	Orif.	Rect.	Lge.	Ind.	0	15	10-15	1-2	
Rheumatism (1)	Pn. Rel.	G-1-P	Lge.	Path.	Lge.	Ind.	0	10-20	15-20	1-2	Mec.
Rheumatism (2)	Pn. Rel.	G-3-P	Lge.	Path.	Lge.	Ind.	0	10	5	2-3	Hist.
Scar tissue	Soften	G-4-N	Med.	Scar	Lge.	Ind.	0	5-15	20-30	2-3	NaCl
Sciatica (1)	N. Sed.	C-1	Lge.	Sc. Notch	Lge.	Calf	15-20	MC	15	3-6	
Sciatica (2)	Pn. Rel.	G-1-P	Lge.	Path.	Lge.	Path.	0	15-20	20	2	Mec.

COND.	AIM	CUR.	ELEC.	PLACE	ELEC.	PLACE	SURGE	INTEN.	TIME	FREQ.	SOLS.
Spider Nevi	Coag.	G-6-N	Needle	Path.	Lge.	Ind.	0	1-3	1-3	1	
Sprains (1)	Decon.	G-P	Med.	Path.	Lge.	Ind.	0	15	15	1-3	
Sprains (2)	Decon.	C-3-4	Med.	Path.	Lge.	Ind.	30	MC	5-10	3-6	
Strictures	Dilate	G-8-N	Orif.	Path.	Lge.	Ind.	0	1-10	5-15	1-2	
Tic douloureux	N. Sed.	G-1-P	Pt.	Path.	Lge.	Ind.	0	10	5-15	1-2	
Tumor	Reduce	G-6-P	Med.	Path.	Lge.	Ind.	0	20	30-40	1	
Ulcers, leg.	Ion.	G-3-P	Pack	Path.	Lge.	Ind.	0	10-15	20	1-3	$CuSO_4$
Uterine sub. inv.	M. Stim.	C-3	Orif.	Vag.	Lge.	Ind.	15	IC	10-15	3-6	
Wry Neck		C-2			Lge.	Ind.	30	IC	5-10	3	

GLOSSARY

Accommodation Change in muscle response to repeated stimuli
Action current Electrical current occurring during the action of muscle or nerve
Action unit Unit current impulse; "spike" potential
Alternating current Current which periodically reverses direction of flow
Ampere The unit of intensity of electric current
Anion An ion carrying a negative charge
Anode The positive pole
Atom The smallest particle of an element
Bipolar The use of two poles in treatment applications
Cable A flexible inductor for applying high frequency energy
Capacitator A device for holding a charge of electricity
Cathode The negative pole
Chronaximetry The measurement of chronaxy
Chronaxy The minimum time at which an impulse of double rheobase intensity will excite contraction
Circuit The course traversed by an electrical current
Closed circuit An active circuit, complete, noninterrupted
Condenser Capacitor
Constant current Unidirectional galvanic current, of constant amplitude
Contractile current Having the power of initiating muscle contraction
Current Flow of electricity of any type
Cycle One complete period of alternating current
d'Arsonval current A high frequency, low voltage current of comparatively high amperage
Denervation Loss of nerve supply
Desiccation The process of drying up
Diathermy Heating of tissues by high frequency energy
Dielectric Insulating substance
Direct current A current that flows in one direction only
Electric massage Massage effects produced by electrical stimulation

Electrocardiogram A graphic tracing of the electric current produced by the contraction of the heart muscle. The normal electrocardiogram shows upward and downward deflections. The first upward deflection, P, is due to the contraction of the auricles. The other deflections are all due to the action of the ventricles

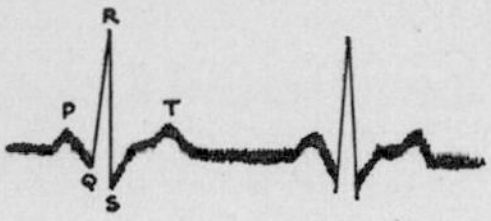

Electrocontractility Contractility in response to electrical stimuli

Electrodiagnosis The use of electricity in diagnosis

Electroencephalogram A graphic record of brain waves

Electrokinetotherapy Multiple muscular stimulation by electrical means

Electron The elemental unit of negative electricity

Electronarcosis Electroshock therapy

Electronic Pertaining to or carrying electrons

Electrolysis Decomposition by means of electricity

Electrolyte A solution capable of conducting electricity

Electromyography The recording of electric potentials of muscles

Electropuncture Electrical stimulation through needles inserted in tissue

Electrotherapy Treatment of disease by means of electricity

Erg The scientific unit of energy

Erythema Abnormal redness of skin

Farad A unit of electrical capacity (very large)

Faradic current A rapid sequence of "spike" impulses

Filter A device for removing ripples from direct current

Franklinic electricity Frictional electricity

Frequency Rate of alternation or recurrence

Fulguration Tissue destruction by sparks

Galvanic current A unidirectional current, unwavering in amplitude

Galvanism Therapeutic application of galvanic current

High frequency Extremely rapid alternations

House current Lighting-supply current

Indifferent electrode The electrode that is not therapeutically active

Induction The production of currents in nonconnected circuits
Innervation Being supplied with nervous energy
Insulator Nonconductor
Ion Any electrically charged particle of matter
Ionization The process of becoming electrically charged
Irritability The ability to respond to stimuli
Joule's law $W = I^2R$
Labile currents Applied by moving electrodes over surface of body
Leduc current Short pulses of direct current with instantaneous "make" and "break"
Leyden jar A two-plate condenser resembling a glass jar
Low frequency Alternations from 1 to 100,000 per second
Low tension Relatively low voltage
Microfarad A unit of capacitance; one millionth of a farad
Microthermy The use of microwaves in thermal therapy
Microwaves Extremely high frequency electromagnetic oscillations
Milliampere Unit of current strength; 1/1000th of an ampere
Monoterminal The use of a single terminal connection
Morton wave current Periodic discharge from a static generator
Motor point Point of greatest response to surface-applied stimuli
Ohm The unit of electrical resistance
Ohm's law $R = E/I$
Open circuit An incomplete electrical pathway; interrupted circuit
Oscillating current A current alternating in direction. When of constant amplitude it is called *undamped*. When it consists of pulses of rapidly diminishing intensity it is called *damped*
Oscilloscope Fluorescent screen for visualization of electrical potential charges
Oudin current A high frequency current of extremely high voltage
Polarity Indication of direction of current flow
Potentiometer Current control device
Primary circuit The circuit connected to power supply
Pulsating current A current varying regularly in intensity
Potential Voltage; electrical pressure

Power Wattage; the rate at which energy is being utilized
Radio frequency Current capable of being radiated
Reaction of degeneration The reaction to electrical stimuli of muscles whose nerves have degenerated
Rectifier Device for changing alternating current to direct current
Resistance Opposition to flow of electrical energy
Resonance The maximum transfer of high frequency energy from one circuit to another
Rheobase The minimum potential of electric current necessary to produce stimulation
Rheostat A variable resistance used to control current flow
Secondary The circuit in which a current is induced
Sensory Pertaining to sensation
Series Connected together, one after the other
Sinusoidal Alternating current of low frequency
Solenoid An inductive coil of wire
Spike A rapidly rising impulse of short duration
Square wave current Sequence of pulses formed by instantaneous make and break of electrical potential
Static current Discharges from a static electricity generator
Static electricity Electricity produced by friction
Superimposed current A rippled direct current; pulsating direct
Surgical diathermy The use of high frequency energy for tissue destruction
Tesla current A high frequency current of medium high voltage
Tetanus Rigid muscular contraction
Thermal current A current used for its heat-producing properties
Threshold Borderline muscular contraction
Transformer A device to change the nature of electrical current
Trigger action A release of energy whose character has no relation to the process which released it
Twitch A single unit of muscular effort
Volt The unit of electromotive pressure
Watt Unit of electrical energy
Wave length Transmission speed divided by frequency

MUSCLE-NERVE TEST CHART NO. 1

Normal Chronaxy Values (Bourguignon)
A-.06-.14 B-.16-.34 C-.36-.70 (Values in Sigma)

PATIENT:
TEST BY:

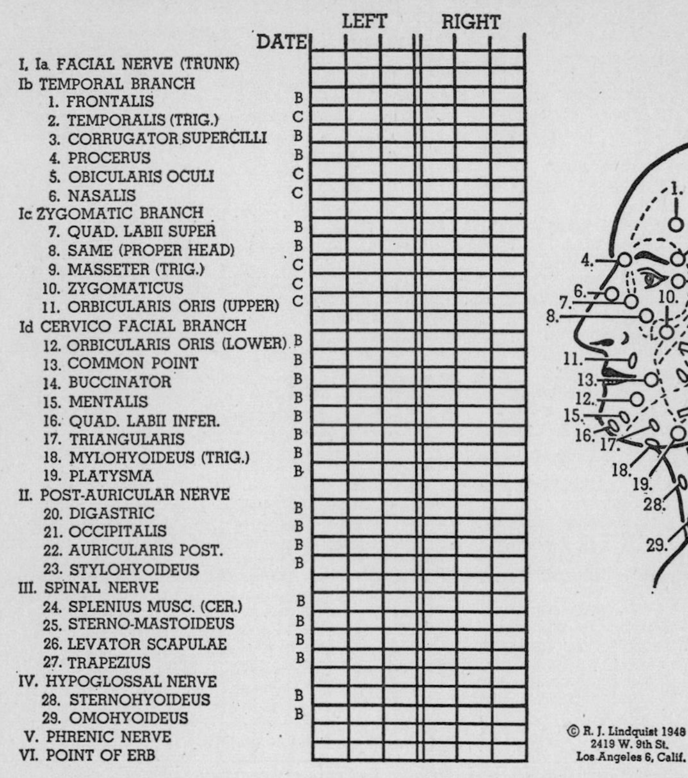

DATE		LEFT			RIGHT		
I, Ia FACIAL NERVE (TRUNK)							
Ib TEMPORAL BRANCH							
1. FRONTALIS	B						
2. TEMPORALIS (TRIG.)	C						
3. CORRUGATOR SUPERCILLI	B						
4. PROCERUS	B						
5. OBICULARIS OCULI	C						
6. NASALIS	C						
Ic ZYGOMATIC BRANCH							
7. QUAD. LABII SUPER	B						
8. SAME (PROPER HEAD)	B						
9. MASSETER (TRIG.)	C						
10. ZYGOMATICUS	C						
11. ORBICULARIS ORIS (UPPER)	C						
Id CERVICO FACIAL BRANCH							
12. ORBICULARIS ORIS (LOWER)	B						
13. COMMON POINT	B						
14. BUCCINATOR	B						
15. MENTALIS	B						
16. QUAD. LABII INFER.	B						
17. TRIANGULARIS	B						
18. MYLOHYOIDEUS (TRIG.)	B						
19. PLATYSMA	B						
II. POST-AURICULAR NERVE							
20. DIGASTRIC	B						
21. OCCIPITALIS	B						
22. AURICULARIS POST.	B						
23. STYLOHYOIDEUS	B						
III. SPINAL NERVE							
24. SPLENIUS MUSC. (CER.)	B						
25. STERNO-MASTOIDEUS	B						
26. LEVATOR SCAPULAE	B						
27. TRAPEZIUS	B						
IV. HYPOGLOSSAL NERVE							
28. STERNOHYOIDEUS	B						
29. OMOHYOIDEUS	B						
V. PHRENIC NERVE							
VI. POINT OF ERB							

FUNCTIONS

1. Raises eyebrows; draws scalp forward.
2. Brings incisors together (elevates the mandible).
3. Draws eyebrows downward and inward.
4. Depresses eyebrow; wrinkles bridge of nose.
5. Closes eyelids.
6. Compresses nostril.
7. Elevates lip; dilates nostril.
8. Proper elevator of upper lip.
9. Muscle of mastication of molars.
10. Elevates lip outward (as in smiling).
11. Sphincter muscle surrounding lips.
12. Closes the mouth.
13. Common point.
14. Compresses cheek, retracts angle of mouth.
15. Raises and protrudes lower lip; wrinkles skin of chin (pouting).
16. Depresses and everts lower lip.
17. Depresses angle of mouth (sorrow).
18. Elevates and advances hyoid.
19. Wrinkles skin and depresses mouth.
20. Elevates hyoid and tongue.
21. Draws scalp backward.
22. Retracts the pinna.
23. Draws hyoid up and back.
24. Extends head and neck, and rotat[e] and flexes laterally.
25. Depresses and rotates head.
26. Elevates upper angle of scapula.
27. Draws head backward.
28. Draws hyoid down (as after swa[l]lowing).
29. Depresses and retracts hyoid.

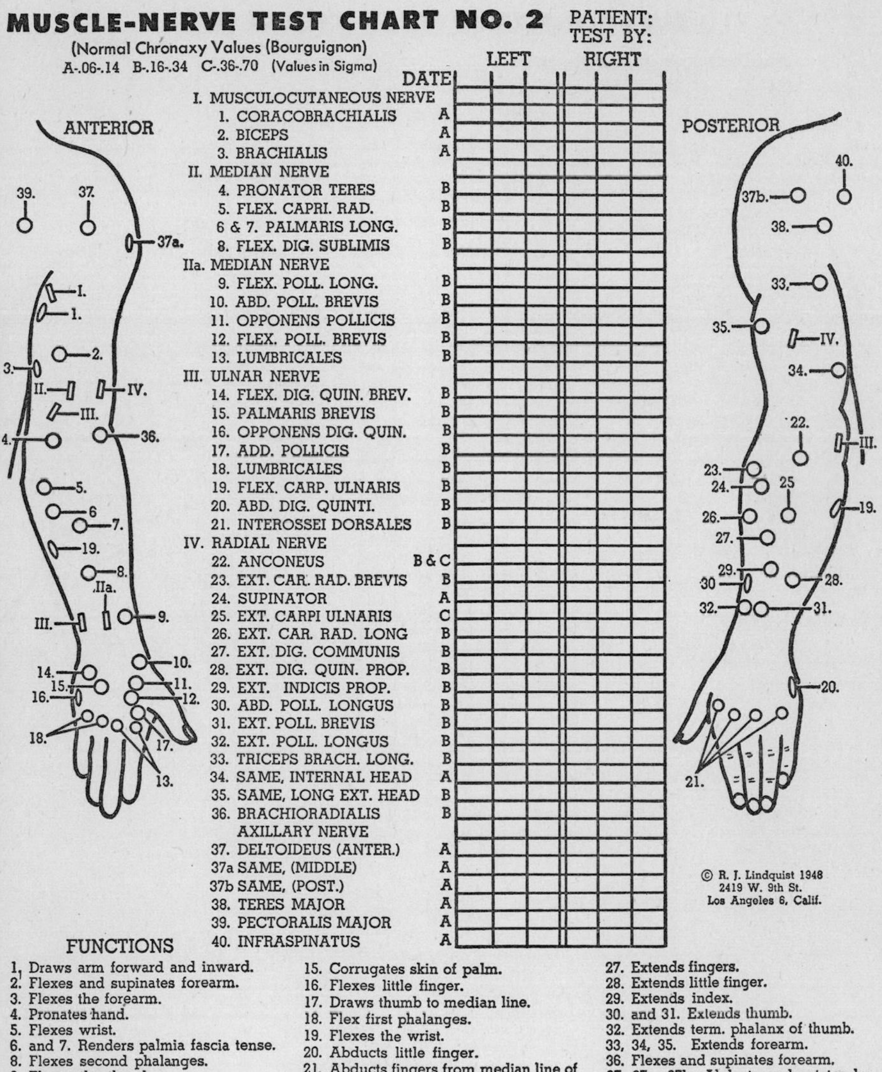

MUSCLE-NERVE TEST CHART NO. 2

PATIENT:
TEST BY:

(Normal Chronaxy Values (Bourguignon)
A-.06-.14 B-.16-.34 C-.36-.70 (Values in Sigma)

DATE		LEFT			RIGHT		
I. MUSCULOCUTANEOUS NERVE							
1. CORACOBRACHIALIS	A						
2. BICEPS	A						
3. BRACHIALIS	A						
II. MEDIAN NERVE							
4. PRONATOR TERES	B						
5. FLEX. CAPRI. RAD.	B						
6 & 7. PALMARIS LONG.	B						
8. FLEX. DIG. SUBLIMIS	B						
IIa. MEDIAN NERVE							
9. FLEX. POLL. LONG.	B						
10. ABD. POLL. BREVIS	B						
11. OPPONENS POLLICIS	B						
12. FLEX. POLL. BREVIS	B						
13. LUMBRICALES	B						
III. ULNAR NERVE							
14. FLEX. DIG. QUIN. BREV.	B						
15. PALMARIS BREVIS	B						
16. OPPONENS DIG. QUIN.	B						
17. ADD. POLLICIS	B						
18. LUMBRICALES	B						
19. FLEX. CARP. ULNARIS	B						
20. ABD. DIG. QUINTI.	B						
21. INTEROSSEI DORSALES	B						
IV. RADIAL NERVE							
22. ANCONEUS	B & C						
23. EXT. CAR. RAD. BREVIS	B						
24. SUPINATOR	A						
25. EXT. CARPI ULNARIS	C						
26. EXT. CAR. RAD. LONG	B						
27. EXT. DIG. COMMUNIS	B						
28. EXT. DIG. QUIN. PROP.	B						
29. EXT. INDICIS PROP.	B						
30. ABD. POLL. LONGUS	B						
31. EXT. POLL. BREVIS	B						
32. EXT. POLL. LONGUS	B						
33. TRICEPS BRACH. LONG.	B						
34. SAME, INTERNAL HEAD	A						
35. SAME, LONG EXT. HEAD	B						
36. BRACHIORADIALIS	B						
AXILLARY NERVE							
37. DELTOIDEUS (ANTER.)	A						
37a SAME, (MIDDLE)	A						
37b SAME, (POST.)	A						
38. TERES MAJOR	A						
39. PECTORALIS MAJOR	A						
40. INFRASPINATUS	A						

FUNCTIONS

1. Draws arm forward and inward.
2. Flexes and supinates forearm.
3. Flexes the forearm.
4. Pronates hand.
5. Flexes wrist.
6. and 7. Renders palmia fascia tense.
8. Flexes second phalanges.
9. Flexes the thumb.
10. Abducts thumb.
11. Flexes thumb.
12. Same, Proximal phalanx.
13. Flex first phalanges.
14. Flexes little finger.
15. Corrugates skin of palm.
16. Flexes little finger.
17. Draws thumb to median line.
18. Flex first phalanges.
19. Flexes the wrist.
20. Abducts little finger.
21. Abducts fingers from median line of middle finger.
22. Extends forearm.
23. Extends wrist.
24. Supinates hand.
25. and 26. Extends wrist.
27. Extends fingers.
28. Extends little finger.
29. Extends index.
30. and 31. Extends thumb.
32. Extends term. phalanx of thumb.
33, 34, 35. Extends forearm.
36. Flexes and supinates forearm.
37, 37a, 37b. Abducts and rotates humerus.
38. Adducts and medially rotates humerus.
39. Draws arm downward and forward.
40. Rotates humerus outward.

MUSCLE-NERVE TEST CHART NO. 3

(Normal Chronaxy Values (Bourguignon)
A-.06-.14 B-.16-.34 C-.36-.70 (Values in Sigma)

PATIENT:
TEST BY:

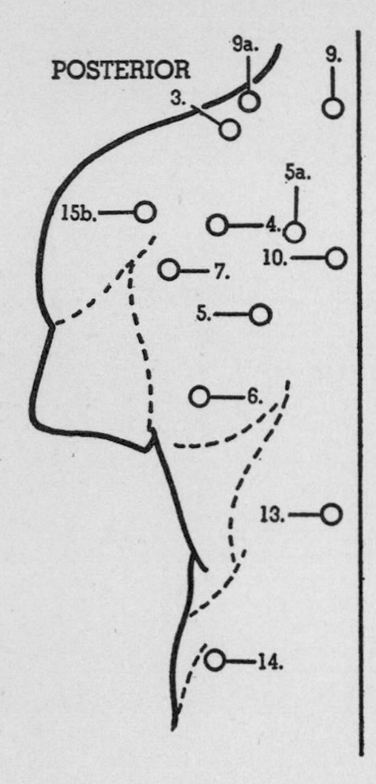

FUNCTIONS

1. Draws arm down and forward.
2. Elevates ribs in inspiration.
3. Supports shoulder joint and raises arm.
4. Rotates humerus outward.
5. Elevates and retracts scapula.
6. Draws arm backward and downward, and rotates inward.
7. Adducts and rotates humerus medially.
8. Depresses the hyoid.
9. Draws head backward.

9a. Same.

10. Same.
11. Compresses viscera and flexes thorax.
12. Same.
13. Extension of spinal column on pelvis: rotation.
14. Rotates, abducts, and advances thigh.
15. 15, 15a, 15b. Abducts and rotates the humerus.

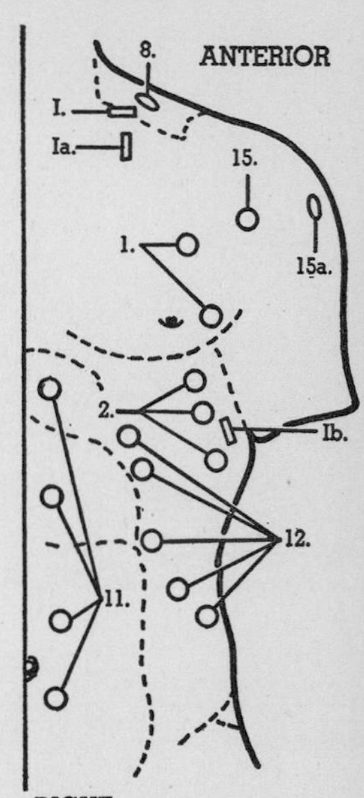

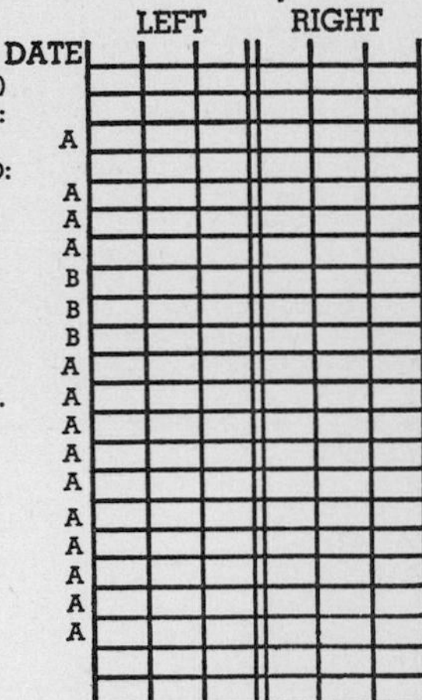

		LEFT			RIGHT		
I. BRACHIAL PLEXUS (POINT OF ERB)							
Ia. ANTERIOR THORACIC NERVE TO:							
1. PECTORALIS MAJOR.	A						
Ib. POSTERIOR THORACIC NERVE TO:							
2. SERRATUS ANTERIOR.	A						
3. SUPRASPINATUS.	A						
4. INFRASPINATUS.	A						
5. RHOMBOID MAJOR.	B						
5a. RHOMBOID MINOR.	B						
6. LATISSIMUS DORSI.	B						
7. TERES MAJOR.	A						
8. STERNOHYOIDEUS (Cerv. Plex.).	A						
9. TRAPEZIUS.	A						
9a. TRAPEZIUS (MIDDLE HEAD).	A						
10. TRAPEZIUS (POST. HEAD).	A						
11. RECTUS ABDOMINIS..	A						
12. OBLIQUUS EXT. ABDOMINIS	A						
13. SACROSPINALIS.	A						
14. GLUTEUS MEDIUS.	A						
15. DELTOIDEUS (ANT.).	A						
15a. Same (MIDDLE).							
15b. Same (POST).							

MUSCLE-NERVE TEST CHART NO. 4

Normal Chronaxy Values (Bourguignon)
A-.06-.14 B-.16-.34 C-.36-.70 (Values in Sigma)

PATIENT:
TEST BY:

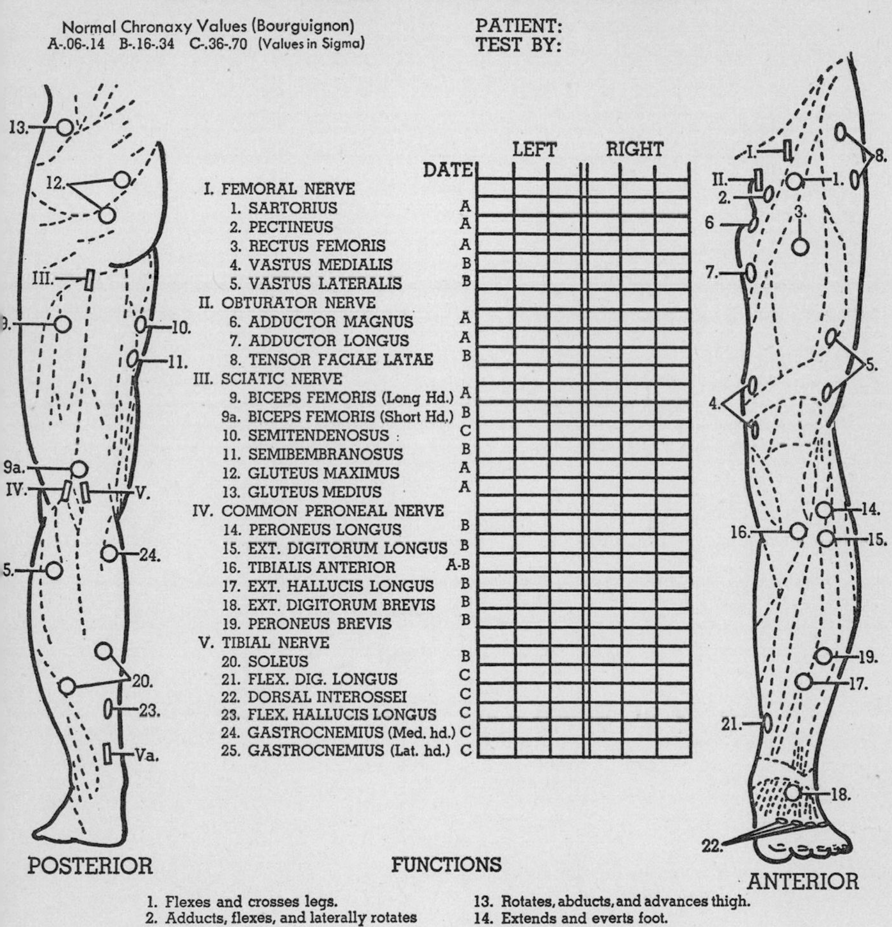

DATE		LEFT	RIGHT
I. FEMORAL NERVE			
1. SARTORIUS	A		
2. PECTINEUS	A		
3. RECTUS FEMORIS	A		
4. VASTUS MEDIALIS	B		
5. VASTUS LATERALIS	B		
II. OBTURATOR NERVE			
6. ADDUCTOR MAGNUS	A		
7. ADDUCTOR LONGUS	A		
8. TENSOR FACIAE LATAE	B		
III. SCIATIC NERVE			
9. BICEPS FEMORIS (Long Hd.)	A		
9a. BICEPS FEMORIS (Short Hd.)	B		
10. SEMITENDENOSUS	C		
11. SEMIBEMBRANOSUS	B		
12. GLUTEUS MAXIMUS	A		
13. GLUTEUS MEDIUS	A		
IV. COMMON PERONEAL NERVE			
14. PERONEUS LONGUS	B		
15. EXT. DIGITORUM LONGUS	B		
16. TIBIALIS ANTERIOR	A-B		
17. EXT. HALLUCIS LONGUS	B		
18. EXT. DIGITORUM BREVIS	B		
19. PERONEUS BREVIS	B		
V. TIBIAL NERVE			
20. SOLEUS	B		
21. FLEX. DIG. LONGUS	C		
22. DORSAL INTEROSSEI	C		
23. FLEX. HALLUCIS LONGUS	C		
24. GASTROCNEMIUS (Med. hd.)	C		
25. GASTROCNEMIUS (Lat. hd.)	C		

FUNCTIONS

1. Flexes and crosses legs.
2. Adducts, flexes, and laterally rotates thigh.
3. Flexes thigh, extends leg.
4. Extends leg and draws patella medially.
5. Extends leg.
6. Adducts and flexes thigh.
7. Adducts thigh and rotates outward.
8. Tenses fascia lata, assists thigh.
9. & 9a. Flexes and rotates leg outward.
10. Extends thigh, flexes leg.
11. Extends thigh, rotates leg inward.
12. Extends, adducts, and draws thigh forward.
13. Rotates, abducts, and advances thigh.
14. Extends and everts foot.
15. Extends toes, dorsiflexes foot.
16. Dorsiflexes foot, inverts it.
17. Extends big toe.
18. Extends toes.
19. Plantarflexes foot, everts it.
20. Plantarflexes foot, steadies leg upon foot.
21. Flexes phalanges, plantarflexes foot.
22. Adduct from middle line of second toe.
23. Flexes big toe.
24. & 25. Extends foot.

CHRONOLOGY OF MUSCLE STIMULATION

1743 d'Helmstadt Suggested that sparks had therapeutic value
1744 Kratzenstein Muscle contraction with static sparks
1745 Musschenbroek Invented Leyden jar
1749 Jollabert Cured paralysis with electric shocks
1750 Nebel Muscular contractions related to electric shocks
1752 Franklin Evolved concept of positive and negative electricity
1786 Galvani Metallic arc stimulation of "animal electricity"
1792 Fabroni Stimulation explained by chemical action
1799 Volta Invention of voltaic pile (direct current stim.)
1825 Nobili Used galvanometer
1825 Sarlandiere Electropuncture needles
1826 Polaprat Galvanic current with electropuncture needles
1827 Ohm Ohm's law
1831 Faraday Discovered that every unit of positive electricity is definitely related to a unit of negative electricity
1832 Henry Self-induction
1837 Addison Static electricity in spasmodic and convulsive diseases
1839 Hall Electricity in differential diagnosis of paralysis
1842 Matteuci Stimulated muscle with faradic current
1848 DuBois-Reymond Stimulus independent of time
1855 Duschenne Localized faradization
1855 Remak Galvanic stimulus applied to motor nerves
1863 Fick Current must have duration to stimulate muscles
1864 Neuman Denervated muscle responds to galvanic, not faradic
1867 Bauche Electrical reaction to crurarized muscles
1867 Erb Described reaction of degeneration
1870 Engleman Determined electrical time constant of muscle
1871 Tiegel Condenser discharge as source of stimulus
1871 Beard and Rockwell General faradization; central galvanization
1872 Chauveau Enunciated laws of contraction
1886 Grutzner Time constant variation among animals and muscles

1888 Tesla Alternating current and induction motor
1889 d'Arsonval Intensity-duration curve
1892 Hoorveg Excitation proven function of time and strength
1897 Thomson Discovered the electron
1899 Waller Optional minimal stimulus
1901 Weiss Ballistic rheotome
1909 Lapicque Definition of chronaxy and rheobase
1912 Bourguignon Chronaxy in man
1934 Monnier Exact formula of electrical excitation
1917 Adrian Mechanism of nervous system
1936 Erlanger and Gasser Electrical signs of nervous activity
1938 A.V. Hill Accommodation of response to stimuli

REFERENCES

HISTORICAL

1875 Beard and Rockwell Medical and Surgical Electricity
1883 Erb Handbook of Electrotherapeutics
1894 Bigelow An International System of Electrotherapeutics
1897 Monell Manual of Static Electricity
1902 Monell The Treatment of Disease by Electric Currents
1912 Coleman Electricity in Diseases of Eye, Ear, Nose, and Throat
1913 Eberhardt High Frequency Manual
1915 Tousey Medical Electricity and X-Rays
1918 Snow High Potential and High Frequency Currents
1918 Sloan Electrotherapy in Gynecology
1920 Neiswanger Electrotherapeutical Practice
1922 Friel Electric Ionization
1926 Cumberbatch Essentials of Medical Electricity
1927 Morgan Electrothermic Methods in Neoplastic Diseases
1927 Sampson Physiotherapy Technic
1928 Dillinger Electrocoagulation of Tonsils
1929 Stewart Physiotherapy
1929 Waddington Practical Index to Electro and Photo Therapy
1929 Garrison History of Medicine

1930 Morse Galvanism and Sine Current Technic
1930 Tovey Copper Ionization in Treatment of Cervicitis
1931 Grover High Frequency Practice

RECENT AND TECHNICAL

1926 Crile A Bi-polar Theory of Living Processes
1928 Adrian The Mechanism of the Nervous System
1932 Newman Chronaxia—Theory and Application to Clinical Neurology
1936 Erlanger and Gasser Electrical Signs of Nervous Activity
1937 Bazzoni Energy and Matter
1937 Kling Histamine Ionization in Rheumatic Conditions
1938 Cross Electricity in Therapeutics
1939 Neussikine and Abramowitz Elektrodiagnostik
1944 Krusen Physical Medicine
1944 Licht The History of Electrodiagnosis
1945 Holmquest and Osborne Technic of Electrotherapy
1945 Kovacs Electrotherapy and Light Therapy
Kovacs Handbook of Physical Therapy
1946 Watkins, et al. Physical Medicine in General Practice
1947 Bierman Physical Medicine in General Practice
1948 Worster Elements of Physical Medicine
1948 Archives of Physical Medicine
1948 Kovacs Yearbook of Physical Medicine

INDEX